ME AND MY PILONIDAL

Little Cyst, Huge Pain In The Ass

Alex Lopez

CONTENTS

DISCLAIMER

This book details the author's personal experiences with and opinions about pilonidals. The author is not a healthcare provider. The information provided in this book is designed to provide helpful information on the subjects discussed. This book is not meant to be used, nor should it be used, to diagnose or treat any medical condition. For diagnosis or treatment of any medical problem, consult your own physician. The publisher and author are not responsible for any specific health or allergy needs that may require medical supervision and are not liable for any damages or negative consequences from any treatment, action, application or preparation, to any person reading or following the information in this book. You understand that this book is not intended as a substitute for consultation with a license healthcare practitioner, such as your physician.

INTRODUCTION

O ver the course of a decade I have lived through five pilonidal cysts. Each one was removed with a surgery, but the stubborn things refused to quit and kept returning. I have dealt with both open and closed wound procedures, and an emergency lancing. These procedures only gave me relief for a few months, or years, before the pilonidal would return again. It was a very frustrating time that kept challenging me physically and mentally. I was pushed to a very low point in my life.

It felt like I was trapped in a constant cycle of pain, relief, and pain again. Everytime I thought I would finally be able to forget about pilonidals I was wrong. I would let my guard down and a burst of pain would signal it's return. I started to live an anxious life. A life where I was scared to sit down, bend over, or lay on my back. If I felt the slightest stiffness or discomfort below my tailbone I would freak out thinking, *oh no, not again!*

Sometimes it was nothing, just my imagination, but during the times that it was a real pilonidal, I knew that there was nothing I could do except go back under the knife and pray that it would be the last time. I hated those moments. The exact second I would realize that I had another pilonidal, everything would freeze. My body would get hot, I would start to stress out, and all I could focus on was the inevitable pain in the ass that was coming to ruin my life. The damn things never had the decency to give me a warning and they never tried to avoid returning during the holidays. It's like they waited for the worst possible times to screw me over. I could be doing absolutely nothing out of the ordinary one moment, and the next minute, I had a volcano erupting from my butt.

It was a miserable time during all those years. But through all that hardship I learned a lot about these cysts, and because of them made long term lifestyle changes, which I believe have decreased my chances of a recurrence. I turned my years of misery into action and learned whatever I could about pilonidals to find different ways of reducing the likelihood that another one would return. I think my efforts over the years, to create new habits and gain new insight into pilonidals, have saved me from the constant pain of these cysts and helped me finally stop the suffering. Instead of wishing for them to go away, or sitting in a pool of my own anxiety, I took it upon myself to help my body keep them away as best it could.

I learned alot about the history, possible causes, and treatment options for pilonidals by doing a lot of digging around for information in different places. A decade ago that was a lot harder to do. It was spread all over the internet and there didn't seem to be clear specific answers on how to solve this problem, only theories and possibilities. But I used what I could and made it work for me. I also had to take an introspective look at myself and take accountability for some of the things I was doing to make the problem worse.

My last operation to remove a pilonidal took place a few years ago, and I don't think that I will be getting another one again. But I still live with the awareness that it can pop up at any moment and send me back under the knife. I am prepared for this, and not anxious or scared about it like I was before. In a way, I'm always going to be ready, and I never let myself forget everything I had to overcome in order to enjoy the life I live now. Regardless of my current mindset, I still understand how difficult this condition can be for everyone who is suffering with it.

Those of us who have dealt with a pilonidal cyst know that this thing hurts the body, and it also affects our mind. The constant shots of pain stop us from thinking coherently and ruin our daily life. A pilonidal can torture and terrify us until we're worn down and unable to do the simplest things. For myself, the pain felt like a hot metal bolt was being pressed towards my tailbone. Bending over, sitting down the wrong way, or even having my pants brush up against it was all it took to feel the pain. I couldn't do anything but freeze and wait for the bolts of agony to fade away. I had to sleep on my side or my stomach every night. Using the toilet and driving both became miserable experiences with the hot metal bolt relentlessly pushing deeper into my tailbone each time.

There's no way to avoid the constant sensation that some kind of pressure is building up underneath. It's enough to make you want to reach back there and tear off your own flesh. If you feel something similar to me then you know how much all of this sucks. But don't give up hope because there's the possibility that it can all go away one day, and if you stay positive, you will have a greater appreciation for your health and your inner strength.

I have written this book for anyone who is new to the world of pilonidals, and those who might be dealing with one all over again and are feeling lost. If this is your first time experiencing this condition, I hope to alleviate some of the stress that comes along with it and prepare you for the road ahead. If you have already experienced a pilonidal, then maybe my stories will feel relatable and the research will give you some new insights into the options available to you for treatment and prevention.

It can be even tougher to deal with it the second or third time around because you know what to expect and feel powerless to stop it. You know that pain is coming. There will be days of discomfort, and eventually some kind of surgery or outpatient procedure to get rid of it. After going through it once we don't look forward to doing it all over again, so just know that it's okay for you to feel like crap during a recurrence.

A pilonidal cyst is brutal. It's many more things than a painful lump. It's annoying, it's stressful, and it constantly beats us down. However, in other ways it also makes us stronger. When you are living your life with a pilonidal cyst, you are overcoming a very difficult experience and through the hardship you can find new strength.

I think in the midst of the pain and suffering your pilonidal has taught you something about yourself. It has shown you that one way or another, you have been pushing forward and trying to survive with this little pain in the ass holding you down. That is amazing in itself because the pilonidal is back there causing problems and stressing you out day and night, but you grit your teeth and don't let it stop you. It takes a strong person to put up with that over and over again. Even if you don't believe it now, I hope you will eventually be able to acknowledge how strong you have been as you deal with this condition.

After overcoming five surgeries, I wish I knew then what I know now, and hope all the details I provide will help you get through this difficult time with less anxiety. The whole process from discovery, to receiving treatment, and post-surgery recovery can feel very confusing. There are a ton of options out there to fix the problem and it's hard to understand what you are getting yourself into until you are actually going through with it. I will try to clarify some of this and make your life a bit easier. If you believe a treatment you have already tried has had no effect I hope to explain some of the possible reasons for that.

It can be hard to find all the information on pilonidals without spending hours on the web. It's scattered in many different places, sometimes it's vague, and other times the specifics can only be found within complicated medical articles. Doctors try to do the best they can to explain the condition, but many aren't able to stay up to date on the latest findings and they stick to what they know and are comfortable with. Some might provide outdated information, or don't explain in detail what is happening in order to help us limit the risk of a recurrence.

For myself, it was only through the lived experience of having multiple pilonidals that I was motivated enough to do some extensive research and learn more about them. It was in response to the sense of helplessness that I took it upon myself to get educated on them. I imagine that you might be in the same position if you are reading this book. You have gotten a ton of different tidbits and want a better idea of what this thing and what to do about it.

I started learning about pilonidal cysts around 2006 when my first bump appeared. It quickly sprung up on the top edge of my ass for no apparent reason. I wasn't worried at that time because it was small and awkwardly located on the very crevice of my butt. It seemed harmless to me, almost like a big pimple. I thought the pain was from some tough workouts that left me with a sore butt. After a couple of doctor visits I realized that it was something much scarier than I could have imagined, and it would be very difficult to deal with. I went through the process of having it diagnosed, treated with antibiotics, and eventually removed with a surgery but that wouldn't be the end of it. The first pilonidal was the start of what would become a long painful journey.

When I dealt with my first pilonidal, I couldn't have believed that I would be going through that same experience four more times. It's ironic that such a small thing could become such a huge pain in the ass. Over the years my pilonidals left me bedridden, and emotionally crippled. Feeling terrified, stressed, anxious, depressed, angry and with a strong sense that I was alone in the struggle.

As the years went by I almost gave up hope. I thought I would suffer for the rest of my life because they kept returning without warning, and for no apparent reason. I seriously started thinking about how to build my life around the occasional surgery. I figured that every year I could use up my vacation days to recover from the surgeries, and instead of traveling or having fun I could spend my time in bed, miserable and alone. But then, after my final pilonidal came and went, with no other recurrences, I felt like a new man. I started to visualize a future where I didn't have to fear this thing anymore. I could be prepared, and take back control. I made the decision to not allow the condition to beat me down again.

Now that I have lived happily for a few years without a recurrence, I can look back and reflect on my whole journey with a new perspective. Each of the recurrences taught me a different lesson about self-care, and how I might have been increasing my risk of a pilonidal. I learned to take care of my body and change my bad habits. I also got a better understanding of how pilonidals come about and how they are treated, which gave me new insight into what was happening below the surface.

To be perfectly honest, it would definitely suck if I developed another pilonidal. I would have to start the process of treatment all over again, but this time I would be better able to manage the experience and not suffocate in my own misery. I am much more prepared for it to happen again, which reduces my stress level and keeps me positive. Maybe it was all thanks to my last surgery that the problem was finally solved, but I also believe that my lifestyle changes have played a huge part in keeping me pilonidal free for the last couple of years, and I want to show you everything I have learned.

The first part of the book will be a breakdown of the medical research on pilonidals. This condition has been getting some attention for many years and over time new procedures have been developed to treat it. I have looked extensively through different medical articles and found information on the different surgery techniques, how they work, and their level of effectiveness. I will breakdown all of that information for a better understanding of pilonidals. Hopefully this can help you understand your options or point you in a certain direction to find out more for yourself.

In the second part, I will share my own personal experience with each of my five cysts. I will describe the hardship and gory details of each one. I will be very honest and very descriptive about what I went through. The entire process from discovery to treatment and recovery was unique for all 5 of the pilondidals. Each one provided me with insights into the mistakes I was making and what I could do differently to prevent recurrences. They were stepping stones to making me a stronger, healthier person, and I think the stories can help you avoid some of my many mistakes.

The third part of the book will be a quick walkthrough of an outpatient excision surgery. I will outline everything that takes place from surgery prep, to the operation, and then recovery. It is broken down into a step by step manner, and will include tips and suggestions that have helped me along the way.

If you are going through this struggle right now, I will reiterate that a pilonidal is absolutely brutal, but it also makes you stronger. I think your pilonidal has taught you something about yourself. You are overcoming a very difficult problem and should take the time to acknowledge the strength you've shown. The fact that you can keep living your life with this little pain in the ass is amazing. Let's get right to it and check out what the research tells us about pilonidal cysts.

UNDERSTANDING PILONIDALS

The existence of this condition has been documented in medical records for at least two centuries. The causes have baffled the medical field ever since it's discovery and have made it very difficult to find the proper method of treatment. Early specialists noted the presence of hairs in a cavity when treating patients who were experiencing pain below their tailbone. They came to a few conclusions based on observations and using the medical technology available to them at the time.

They believed that hairs would become trapped inside a tiny cavity around the natal cleft, which is basically the deep groove between your butt cheeks. It was argued that these hairs would lead to the formation of a sinus, which is a small tunnel or hole in the skin. The sinus would grow larger if left untreated, and could often develop into an infected abscess.

As a result, the term pilonidal was created by combining the Latin terms pilus, a hair, and nidus, a nest (Jain & Thambuchetty, 2016). For a long time this was the only root cause that doctors could point to as the source of pilonidals. Anyone with a painful bump at the top of their cleft would get it checked out by a doctor who would usually find some type of trapped debris inside like hair follicles. The debris would be cleared out and it appeared that as a result the problem should have been fixed. Unfortunately that wasn't how things went.

The answer seemed simple. Doctors would basically cut into the patient to clean out hair and debris from the sinus, and then send them on their way. The people would be left with sore butts and not much else to worry about. It helped them find some relief for a while, but eventually many of them started to return multiple times for the same treatment. It became clear that the problem was more complicated than doctors initially believed, and they would quickly realize that a simple incision and cleaning of the area would not be enough to fix it everytime.

This must have been very frustrating for early pilonidal patients because there was no second option. It was only after multiple recurrences were documented, over and over again, with different patients that doctors began to search for more solutions. But before that happened many more people would have to be diagnosed with pilonidals to demonstrate there was a large enough need for new treatments.

During World War II there was an increasing interest in the condition when it was frequently diagnosed among soldiers. It was labeled "the jeep disease" because it mostly affected jeep drivers. These troops spent a lot of time traveling over rough terrain on top of very stiff seats. The vehicles weren't built for comfort and their butts had to absorb a lot of the impact.

This time around some specialists believed that the constant bouncing on the seat, as they drove through rocky roads, led to regular trauma to the tailbone and eventually a pilonidal. The evidence was not conclusive enough for this to be determined as the main cause, but it brought another potential factor into play.

For many soldiers this was their first pilonidal, and treatment options hadn't changed much since earlier times. They would have their pilonidal cut open, cleaned out, and closed up in order to send them back out into the field. I have a belief that these cases might have fed into a false notion that this was not a serious condition. I would imagine some specialist may have thought that the treatments available at the time were good enough because all the soldiers receiving them were able to get back into the fight pretty quickly after surgery. I think this would limit how much time and energy was being put into coming up with new treatments.

Fortunately, some research did continue in the following decades up until present day, and it has answered a lot of the unknowns about pilonidals. Providing a clearer picture of the causes, and improving the level of treatment beyond what many pilonidal patients had to endure in previous times. Here is what researchers have been able to find.

Pilonidal sinuses affect, on average, 26 out of every 100,000 people (Jain & Thambuchetty, 2016). With numbers like that it is possible that you have met someone who has suffered with pilonidals, but you might not know it because a ton of people don't want to talk about it when they have one. This was definitely something I could relate to. The first few times I felt ashamed of having a pilonidal and didn't want anyone to find out.

Men suffer from pilonidals at a higher rate than women (Jain & Thambuchetty, 2016). This might be due to various factors that we will discuss later on. The age group at highest risk falls between 17 to 40 years old. That is a huge range, but even people younger than 17 and older than 40 can get their first pilonidal. With statistics like these it almost feels like no one is free from the risk. I was around 17 when I experienced my first one, and the last one was around 27. Currently at 32 years old, I am still at high risk of a recurrence for the next decade and possibly longer. That is something that I definitely keep in the back of my mind.

As we learned more about pilonidals a few different terms were created to describe them. Each name relates to a different aspect of the condition. In the earlier stages it is known as a pilonidal sinus. This is when a pilonidal first forms a sinus, or tract, which is the small tunnel that develops under the skin when something like a hair burrows into the body. Small pits can also form when the skin is stretched repeatedly, or bruised in some way that damages the hair follicles. A sinus can be very small and almost undetectable to the human eye, making it hard to catch early on. Also, since they appear around the top crease of the butt, we can never really look at the area closely, increasing the difficulty of detecting them.

A sinus can appear harmless and usually does not result in any pain at first. Also, it is possible to have some debris penetrate the skin without developing a sinus. There might have been times when we were on the verge of getting one and never even realized it. If the body can push out the object, or heal the tract, then everything should remain normal.

On top of that, trauma or constant pressure also won't always develop a sinus. But the moment a sinus does develop, regardless of the cause, a pilonidal is officially present. For that reason we can think of this as the initial stage of a pilonidal. If it doesn't develop past this phase then it might go away on its own, or maybe remain dormant for a long time. It is possible to have a sinus long before you realize it. It can be there not doing much and your body won't alert you that anything is wrong.

When this small tunnel, or hole, gets filled with debris, it can become a pilonidal cyst. This is the sac that forms at the top of the butt, and is often times the first visible sign of a pilonidal. Many people notice that something is wrong when the cyst comes along, not realizing that it has likely been developing underneath the skin for a while.

This makes it hard to pinpoint an exact moment that may have caused a pilonidal to spring up. Some people say they remember developing a pilonidal shortly after injuring their tailbone. It is possible that the injury was the source of their pilonidal, but it could have also been countless other things that they do everyday.

Think back to the days and weeks before you noticed your pilonidal, I am sure you can think of a ton of things you were doing like sitting down, laying on your back, working out, or going on a long car ride that might have increased your risk for a pilonidal. Maybe your clothes were on too tight and rubbed you the wrong way at the wrong time. Who knows, the cleft of your butt might have been stretched a few too many times and decided that it was the time to start causing some problems, and got things moving in the wrong direction.

Much like the sinus, you can have a cyst and not experience any pain which makes it easy for many people to notice it at first, and then try to ignore it. They will delay medical treatment because it's one of those things that seems to go away on its own. It is possible that it could disappear even at this stage, but the likelihood is very small and growing increasingly smaller. It may only go dormant and shrink in size before returning.

However, if the sinus, or the cyst that follows becomes infected, a pilonidal abscess can form. When this happens the area might become painful and grow larger or more pointed at the top as if pressure is building up underneath. It can also leak pus or blood at different stages, but that is most likely to start after an infection because the body is trying to clear out all the debris and fix the problem.

Even though a pilonidal can be more specifically identified as a sinus, cyst, or abscess, most doctors and patients will probably call it a pilonidal cyst for the sake of keeping things simple. When I talk about a pilonidal cyst I am usually referring to the infected bump.

By the time the pilonidal cyst comes around the symptoms can vary from person to person. Some may experience no pain at all, and for others it can be excruciating. We can look in the mirror one day and all of a sudden see a swollen cyst that is already infected. That can be a shocking sight, but at least it lets us know that something is wrong. If that inflamed cyst starts leaking fluid, well for one that can be embarrassing, but two it also tricks us into thinking that it has popped and will soon go away. The cyst can shrink after releasing the buildup and bring a sense of relief. The pain might fade away and the area will look like it's going back to normal. Unfortunately, it can start to grow again and be right back to its swollen state within days.

The cyst can also drain, but not shrink at all and continue to remain painful. In those situations the drainage brings no relief, not even momentarily. I had one of those in my time. It kept leaking daily, the size wouldn't decrease and the pain was always there. I took antibiotics which only numbed it temporarily and slowed down the leaking, but never really stopped it. The pain and swelling came back as soon as the antibiotics ran out and I was right back where I started. This is the worst point of the pilonidal, and ideally you never want it to get that bad.

Possible Causes

Although nothing conclusive has been found regarding the causes of pilonidals, research has given us a better understanding of the condition. It is not believed to be an acquired disease, which means it's not likely that your parents passed it down to you. This might sound surprising to some of you, especially if you have family members who have dealt with pilonidals. Since it affects millions of people all over the world, it's likely that you will know someone who has had it, and your family history might be riddled with a few pilonidal occurrences.

There are some factors that may predispose people, such as myself, to this disease and increase the chances of developing it. These factors include; having a deep natal cleft, experiencing trauma to the area, obesity, or a sedentary life with long periods of sitting, and excessive hair in the area (Yoldas, et al., 2013). Each of these might increase the chances of developing a pilonidal sinus by allowing a hair follicle, or other debris, to burrow into the skin. Or they can create the conditions for a sinus to form without any penetrating debris by simply causing trauma to the flesh and skin in the area.

These factors shouldnt be taken as an indication that everyone who can check them off will develop a pilonidal. Millions of people can sit on their butt all day, have poor hygiene, a hairy butt, and so on, but never even get close to developing a pilonidal.

For those of us that do end up with a pilonidal, it might start with the penetration of a hair follicle into the skin. In order for that to happen there must be a force that causes the insertion, and also vulnerable skin to allow access (Jain & Thambuchetty, 2016). Let's look at an example to explain how you might develop a pilonidal from some hair follicles.

Imagine it's a regular weekday and you are working at a desk job or in a classroom. You are spending countless hours sitting down on a stiff chair. Day after day you sit on your butt with some bad posture, constantly readjusting on your chair to get more comfortable. With these small adjustments you keep bumping and grinding on your butt. The movements are constant and you do it without really noticing. You have some hair around your butt, and one super tiny follicle falls into the natal cleft.

With the constant shuffling you keep pressing and grinding the area around your tailbone. Throw in some bad posture on top of that, and you have created better conditions for the fallen hair follicle to burrow into your tender stretched out skin. The follicle works its way inside and forms a tiny sinus. You now have the initial stage of what could become a pilonidal cyst.

By comparison, someone who spends more time on their feet and is fairly hairless down there would decrease the chances of having that same scenario play out. It doesn't mean they won't develop a pilonidal, but the risk is reduced. Their tailbone is freed from hours of pressure, and without hair a follicle is less likely to create a cavity. If there is an opportunity to reduce the risk of a pilonidal by making lifestyle changes then I believe it is worth the effort.

Taking time to stand up, use a coccyx cushion, and shave could be small actions with huge benefits in the long run. It's really a matter of taking a look at your situation as you sit down and asking, if you can do more to take care of your butt.

The previous example is not the only method for a sinus to form. If you receive regular trauma to the area through activities like driving, boating, and exercising it could potentially lead to the development of a sinus. Something as simple as situps on the hard ground can stretch and grind the skin enough to damage hair follicles. You can even have some debris buildup from sweating as you go about your busy life. The excessive moisture allowing things to remain trapped in the cleft and increasing your level of risk. Even a random injury that bruises your tailbone can be the start of everything. Keep in mind these are not all the potential culprits, and this don't include some of the internal mechanisms that we will discuss further on.

With the root cause of pilonidals being so difficult to

pinpoint, different treatments have been created to address various factors. The simple incision, drainage, and cleaning of the area that was commonly used before often failed to prevent a recurrence and it became evident to specialists that pilonidals were more complicated than they initially believed. It would take more than cleaning out a nest of hairs to cure patients. Surgeons started to take more factors into account and updated their strategies to improve upon the success rate of treatments.

In recent decades doctors have tried to cure patients by focusing on 3 different aspects of the condition, the sinus, the cleft of the butt, and postoperative healing. By addressing these three things it is believed that the chances of a recurrence can be reduced.

First, the sinus is the small tunnel or hole that can form inside the skin and bring about a pilonidal. It is the first sign of a problem that can lead to an abscess or cyst. Dealing with it early on can potentially make for an easier operation and recovery.

After one of my closed wound surgery procedures I noticed the sinus very qucikly when a tiny piece of stitching was protruding from my skin right in the middle of my fresh scar. The doctor had previously said it wasn't necessary to remove the stitches because they would be absorbed into my body during the healing process. Well that didn't happen, and I believe it left just enough space for a tiny hole to form. I went on to have another pilonidal shortly after that. But this time I noticed it early on and rushed to the doctor at the very first sign of a bump.

The surgery and recovery that followed were a lot easier because we took care of it quickly and there was only one sinus to deal with. This emphasizes the importance of detecting the sinuses quickly and removing all the sinuses during a treatment. It can have a huge impact on future pilonidal risk.

Second, the cleft of the butt is problematic because of its depth, curvature, and the constant pressure and trauma it has to endure. By making changes to that area it might be possible to reduce the likelihood of another pilonidal popping up. If we can smoothen it out then a pilonidal will have less than ideal conditions to develop within a shallower cleft. Later on we will discuss a popular treatment that makes changes to the cleft of the butt.

Finally, a third aspect of the condition that new treatments try to work on is postoperative healing. Proper wound care can have a huge impact on the rate of recurrence. By keeping our wound clean after surgery we reduce debris build up and prevent infections in the new tissue. Infections and debris can support the conditions for a pilonidal to form and we want to avoid them at all cost. Unfortunately that can be hard to do when it comes to wounds. Especially when it is located right in the crevice or our butt. Even a few careless moments can lead to trouble. Some of the treatment options we will discuss also try to increase our chances of success during wound healing by making it easier to manage the stitches from surgery.

I will now cover a few of the different techniques that have been created to treat pilonidal cysts, and also present the results of research examining their effectiveness. As you will read, some of the treatment options attempt to do more than clear out the debris, and actually make an effort to address the sinus, the cleft of the butt, and post-operation healing. They have improved over time, but most still require a surgical procedure.

TREATMENT OPTIONS

There are many different options for removing a pilonidal, the majority of them involving surgery. As you will see, over time some have improved upon their predecessors and the success rate has at least continuously improved.

Incision And Drainage

One of the quickest and most manageable treatments is an incision and drainage, sometimes known as a lancing. This procedure is very common and can be the fastest way to relieve the pain of an infected cyst. It has been around for a long time and most doctors know how to do it, even if they aren't experts on pilonidal cysts. The whole procedure is also more affordable and accessible to the general public. Most hospitals and emergency rooms can do it with only local anesthesia, which means you are not completely put to sleep.

With this treatment you have to lay face down and the area around your butt is injected with anesthetic to numb it. The injection is meant to reduce sensation, but unfortunately you will still feel pain because localized anesthetic can't completely stop the pain from registering. After a few moments the doctor makes a cut to open up and drain the cyst. That initial slice is quick but it hurts alot. The doctor then presses the sides of the cyst together to force out all the fluid inside. As the blood and pus flow out a small machine might be used to suck it all up before it gets too messy. Once the pus and debris is pushed out the pain of the pilonidal disappears. Gauze (surgical dressing) is packed into the small wound that is leftover to stop the bleeding and the procedure is done.

The gauze keeps the wound free of debris as it heals. The wound will not be too deep and it won't require too much post-treatment care. The whole process doesn't take more than a few minutes after the numbing agent is injected. Patients are left with a sore butt, and after a few minutes of lying down to recover, they can walk out of the hospital and go about their life. The wound will close up within a couple of days and the gauze will no longer be needed.

Incision and drainage has one of the higher rates of recurrence because multiple sinuses can be missed and some debris can remain trapped. The doctor can only make a shallow cut and it is not enough to get a good look at the whole pilonidal down to the root. The cut only cleans out the infection and debris but does not do enough to the sinuses. If you have multiple tracts, then it's possible that they can develop into a cyst or abscess pretty quickly after the treatment. One sinus with a deep tunnel, that can't be fully reached by the incision, will lay dormant for a while until a build up of debris brings about another cyst.

On the positive side, this treatment can provide immediate

relief for anyone with a painful cyst that is having trouble doing simple day to day stuff. It can get you back to work faster, or even provide some relief before a surgery that might be scheduled for a later time.

This treatment is often used for those people who are experiencing their first pilonidal and with only one noticeable sinus. A doctor might not find it necessary to do a full blown surgery if there is a chance that the pilonidal will go away after an incision and drainage. Sometimes they want to avoid causing trauma and hardship to a patient until they have tried a less invasive option.

The one thing to keep in mind is that an incision and drainage can get you back on your feet faster than most other treatments, but it will hurt, and your recurrence rate might be higher. This trade off is something that you can discuss with your doctor and base it on your specific situation. However, even though the procedure is painful, it feels amazing to get rid of the fluid build up. I received this treatment in an emergency room when one of my pilonidals felt like a hot volcano that wouldn't erupt. It was so painful that I was barely able to walk. I felt feverish and in complete agony until this procedure finally saved me from the misery.

Open/Closed Wound Excision

Another treatment technique is open/closed wound excision. This is an outpatient procedure which means it can take a few hours to complete and the patient has to be put to sleep. This treatment is much more intensive than the incision and drainage because it requires that a large piece of flesh be cut out to remove the pilonidal sinus, not just clear out the debris. The distinction between open and closed excision is based on the type of wound that is left after surgery. The surgical procedure itself is similar for both.

During an excision, the patient will need to spend a few hours in the hospital. This can't be done in a regular doctor's office since it is more intensive, and requires a team of medical professionals to help the surgeon.

First, an IV is inserted to administer anesthesia. Within seconds the patient will be asleep and have no idea what is happening as they are taken into an operating room. The surgeon and medical team then cut out a large chunk of flesh around the pilonidal to completely remove the sinus, and tracts. By being able to cut in deeper and wider than a regular incision, they can remove multiple sinuses and get to the bottom of any long tracts.

The exact size and depth of the wound will vary from person to person. The surgeon won't really know themselves how much flesh needs to be cut out until they are in the operating room. On the outside a pilonidal might look small, but it's roots can run deep. After the surgery the patient slowly wakes up in a recovery room where they are observed for about 30-45 minutes. They aren't released until they are fully conscious and can use the bathroom on their own. At this point the patient might be informed if they have to deal with a primary closed wound, or a secondary open wound.

In primary closure, the wound is stitched up along the midline of the butt, right along the crevice. The top layer of skin is closed while the flesh underneath is still healing. Over the course of a few weeks new tissue will form, and ideally there will be no more pilonidal sinuses. The risk with this healing process lies in the possibility of having tiny gaps within the newly formed tissue. As your body heals, those tiny spaces might increase the risk of another pilonidal.

Once the stitches are used to seal up the excision there is not much else you can do other than wait and hope that proper wound care above the skin reduces the likelihood of developing a sinus. A focused effort needs to be made to keep the skin above and around the stitches very clean and protected at all times.

With secondary, open wound healing, the wound is left open after the pilonidal is removed. You have to care for it until it fully heals up and closes on its own. The open wound will require you to fill it up with gauze to prevent the outer edges from touching or debris from falling in. The objective is for the bottom tissue to heal first and have everything seal shut from the bottom up. This will hopefully prevent any empty spaces or tiny gaps from forming inside because we are not forcing the two sides of the wound to merge together.

The gauze has to be changed on a daily basis. It has to be pulled out, and fresh gauze has to be pushed in. The wound slowly becomes more shallow, and day by day less gauze needs to be packed inside. As you can see, unlike the closed wound it attempts to reduce the probability of gaps forming and minimizes the probability of developing another sinus. There is still some debate whether this open wound technique actually works better at reducing the risk in comparison to closed wound.

Primary closed wound has a faster healing time and requires a lot less maintenance because it uses stitches. But, there is evidence that secondary open wound healing has a lower rate of recurrence, and it is more often used for those patients who can't get rid of their pilonidal with the first surgery. The effectiveness of one over the other hasn't been completely proven, but some research has drawn some interesting comparisons.

Hosseini et al. (2006) conducted a study on these two procedures. They took 80 patients with a pilonidal abscess and separated them into two groups. Group A received a drainage treatment followed by an excision surgery 3 weeks later with primary closure (closed wound). Group B had an excision with secondary healing (open wound). The same surgeon operated on all the patients.

The researchers compared the groups on wound healing, postoperative complications, and signs of recurrence for 12 months after the surgery. The results showed that all the patients were back to work within 7-9 days, with no signs of recurrence in the following 6 months. After 12 months, 14% of the people in group A (closed wound) experienced a recurrence, and there were no recurrences in group B at that time (Hosseini, et al., 2016). The infection rate for group A was 5.6%, and 2.5% for group B (Hosseini, et al., 2016). As a result, the authors would not recommend primary closure for more severe cases of pilonidal abscesses, due to the recurrence rate. (Hosseini, et al., 2016). The closed wound procedure might be good for anyone on their first pilonidal, but they don't recommend it after that.

In another study, Fahrni et al. (2016) found excision, with

secondary open wound healing, to be the preferable method of treatment because the excision with stitches down the midline had a high recurrence rate. Even though open wound excisions have a lower recurrence rate, in comparison to midline closures, they do have a longer postoperative recovery period. The median recovery time being about 5.4 weeks for open wounds (Yoldas, et al., 2013).

After one of my closed wound procedures I was able to return to work within a week and a half, but I did experience pain above my stitches and could only sit and work for about 4 hours at a time. In comparison, after an open wound procedure I had a doctor tell me that I could do anything from hiking to riding a horse right away with no problem. I was very surprised to hear that because the wound was large and deep. He definitely downplayed the severity of it. I didn't feel confident leaving my house until about 1 month after the surgery, and needed nearly 2 months before that wound completely closed up.

It seems like we can return to normal life pretty quickly, but in my experience, I think it's better to let the body heal as long as possible in order to be on the safe side. That can be hard to do. It's not easy to take extra time from work or school, and there are a lot of other responsibilities that pressure us to get back to business as usual. We can deal with minor pain and suck it up, but that doesn't mean we should. If there are ways to extend our healing time I think it's worth it.

The biggest difference between these two treatment options might come down to the post-operation healing process. The open wound procedure requires time, patience, and some helping hands for the constant gauze changes. In exchange it might reduce the chances of a recurrence. The closed wound will be quicker, and easier to manage, but could come with an increased risk of recurrence, although that has not been confirmed.

With all that in mind, it is possible that a closed wound excision can be recommended to treat the first pilonidal a person experiences. Especially if it is discovered early and before any infection sets in. First time patients may not be high risk for a recurrence, and may not have to worry about dealing with it again. This would make the closed wound ideal to get them back to normal life a bit faster with less hassle.

Pilonidal patients should be able to discuss these two options with their surgeon before receiving treament, but many are never given the pros and cons or an option to choose. In my experience, I was never asked if I preferred one or the other. The surgeon only gave me a vague explanation of what I might expect and that was the end of it. I think that even if I did know enough to ask the right questions, my doctor would not have been able to tell me if the wound would be left open or closed until he got a look at the situation in the operating room.

After my surgeries I wouldn't find out what type of wound I had until I got home, removed the bandages, and looked in the mirror. The moment the top layers of gauze came off I would either be staring at a row of stitches, or the inside of my body.

It also never occurred to me to ask about my options because I didn't know that there were different techniques available. This highlights a rarely discussed problem when seeking treatment for pilonidals, the lack of patient input.

Many medical professionals suggest the use of open or closed wound excision. But the decision to use one or the other is usually made by the surgeon without discussing it with the patient and when they are already on the operating table. That makes it very hard to prepare for recovery. Healing time, pain levels, and risk of recurrence are all impacted by the decisions the surgeon makes in the operating room and it can be frustrating to be kept out of the loop until we are already home post-surgery. To avoid that problem I think we should all feel empowered to ask more questions about treatment options, and find surgeons who are well-informed on different surgical procedures.

The incision and drainage, along with open and closed wound excisions are usually the first treatment options that many of us experience. They can be like the entry points. If no more pilonidals come after that then we are basically done even though the risk of another one can remain for many years. For those of us unfortunate enough to get a second pilonidal, we end up looking for more options.

Flap and Cleft Procedures

Even with the improvements made by the open and closed wound surgeries the likelihood of developing another pilonidal remained high for people all over the world, and over the years specialist have tried to develop better techniques for positive long term results. After attempting to address the sinuses with excisions, the cleft and crevice of the butt became the big focus for new treatments. That area seemed to be a potential culprit for the high recurrence rate.

We can all have different shaped clefts, with some being deeper or wider than others. After a surgery, a deeper cleft could increase the chances of building up debris and forming another pilonidal even if all the sinuses are removed. Furthermore having stitches right down the crevice can create the conditions for poor wound care and another recurrence. This hasn't been found to be a definitive cause, but in the search for new solutions specialists worked on procedures that would avoid leaving a patient with stitches and wounds down the midline of the butt (Pappas & Christodoulou, 2018).

Different techniques utilizing flaps have been developed to move the sutures away from the midline and avoid issues with the crevice of the butt (Aithal, Rajan, & Reddy, 2012). By moving the stitches away from the midline and onto the buttcheeks, there is less risk for infection and debris build up. Flap techniques allow for the surgeons to control the location of the stitches and improve the success rate of closed wounds.

Specialists have also tried to find ways to reshape and level out a patient's cleft to make it more shallow. A shallower cleft helps reduce the potential risk for another pilonidal. With these new techniques a surgeon could deal with two more risk factors by reshaping the cleft, and moving the stitches away from the crevice.

Some of the treatments developed to move stitches away from the midline include Z-plasty, Karydakis flap, and Limberg flap (Pappas & Christodoulou, 2018). There is also the Bascom Cleft Lift which has been standing out from the crowd in recent years, and we will go into more detail on what sets it apart later on. The goal of these procedures is to help the pilonidal sufferers maintain good hygiene because they won't have to deal with stitches right down their crevice. It makes it easier to clean themselves after using the bathroom or while showering. They not only eradicate the sinus, but also get rid of another of the other factors responsible for sinuses developing (Jain & Thambuchetty, 2016).

Two of the more popular surgeries utilizing these improved strategies include the Karydakis, and Limberg flap procedures. These are both outpatient procedures that require you to be put to sleep while the pilonidal sinus is removed similar to the open/closed excision previously discussed. They can take a few hours to complete and will leave you feeling beat up just like the open and closed wound surgeries. These procedures keep the wound closed, there is no open wound option due to the complicated stitches that need to be put in place.

A study conducted by Bali, et al. (2015) examined 71 patients from 2009-2013 with recurrent pilonidal sinus, who were treated with Limberg flap and Karydakis flap. They found that the Limberg technique had a lower complication rate, shorter hospital stay, lower pain experienced, and higher patient satisfaction (Bali, et al., 2015).

One concern with these procedures is the extra amount of stitches that are needed to move the wound away from the midline which could result in a longer scar. Let me try to break down the Limberg flap and explain why more stitches are needed to close this wound.

During the procedure they cut out a chunk of flesh right

around the top of your butt where the pilonidal is located. Next, another wound is opened up to the right of that first excision. They take the skin and tissue that is between those two excisions, and pull it over to the left, to close up the first wound and seal it shut with stitches. The flesh around the second cut is then pressed together and also closed up with stitches. You are left with sutures across your butt cheek that almost spell out the letter N. The stitches are not directly over the butt crack and instead move away from the tailbone. A scar will then form above those stitches.

You can easily find images online that give you an idea of what the stitches and scar will look like, but be careful about going down that rabbit hole. A lot of times the pics that get the most clicks receive the top spots in the search results, and those are probably coming from extreme examples of scars and stitches. Over time any scaring should fade away, never completely gone, but much less visible. I am not mentioning the N shaped stitches from the Limberg flap to scare you away from the procedure, but to let you know that you should feel comfortable asking about details like this for any surgery you get.

I have a scar from all my open and closed wound surgeries and no one ever explained to me what to expect. I remember it as being something I was really worried about early on. After 5 surgeries my scar is noticeable, but doesn't make my butt look terrible. It starts about 1 inch above my cleft and runs down the midline of my butt in a straight line. It is mostly on one buttcheek and is only around ½ wide. There is a bit of a wrinkle to it and it's slightly indented, but I don't mind it.

The good thing is that each surgery did not make it much larger. I actually thought that at one point my body would give up and stop trying to heal in that area from all the trauma, but I discovered how resilient the tissue can be. Once I got comfortable letting significant others see it I never heard any complaints, so don't let all of this freak you out.

One of the more popular techniques that not only moves the stitches away from the crevice, but also works to reshape the cleft, is the Bascom Cleft Lift. The goal of this procedure, in reshaping the cleft, is to create a shallow and well-aerated environment for the wound. By reducing the depth of the cleft it makes it harder for moisture or debris to build up.

A study following 127 patients that received this treatment found that only 3 patients reported a recurrence after 1-year (Yoldas, et al., 2013). The recurrence rate for the Bascom procedure has been shown to be as low as 8%. That's much better than the average that has been found by some studies for other techniques like the closed wound procedure. People with multiple sinuses or recurrences have successfully used this technique to finally put an end to their condition. Word has been getting around about the success rate and it is growing in popularity. It's probable that you will find many people discussing it on forums and social media.

The Bascom Cleft Lift is similar to the Karydakis and Limberg procedures. The patient is put to sleep and an excision is made to remove the sinus. It takes a few hours to complete and requires a team of specialists. After any pilonidal sinuses are removed, stitches are used internally to make some changes to the cleft. This is an important component of the surgery because it is the moment that the surgeon can reduce the depth of the cleft. Once they are done the wound is closed up with stitches that move away from the midline, instead of directly above the crevice. As mentioned before this is to improve cleanliness and avoid debris buildup.

A drain might be inserted to help remove any internal fluid buildup, and that is removed about 2-5 days post-surgery. Recovery times vary, but it might be about 14 days until the patient feels functionally normal. However, it is about 6 weeks or more before they feel comfortable enough to lift things and do some physical activities.

The Bascom Cleft Lift is unfortunately not universally used by all surgeons who work with pilondals. It may be hard to find a surgeon in your area who can do it, and the treatment will likely be more expensive than other options. If you want to find a doctor to perform the Bascom Cleft Lift, then a great place to look is on Reddit or Facebook groups where pilonidal survivors can inform you of any specialist they might know. Even with this procedure a recurrence is not impossible, but for those who have tried other options, this could be the next logical step.

When deciding if you want to get one of these various flap procedures, you may have to consider the cost, and your willingness to travel for the operation. If there is no specialist in your area then you might need to do a long car ride, or take a flight, and stay in another city. On the positive side post-operation care is easier since it doesn't leave you with an open wound, and the stitches are not right above your buttcrack. Also, the possibility of having a lower rate of recurrence can be a blessing for those who have dealt with multiple pilonidals.

For those of you concerned about the cosmetic results of an operation, there are less invasive procedures including phenol treatments, and laser depilation. These are primarily used with the first pilonidal that a person experiences because other treatments such as flap reconstruction or open wound excision might be recommended to manage recurrences (Yoldas, et al., 2013).

With phenol treatments, a chemical is injected into the sinus on a regular basis to treat it. The liquid is allowed to flow into the tracts and sit for a few minutes until it is removed by the doctor. This is minimally invasive, but may not be effective with more serious cases of pilonidal cyst, or abscesses, until they are excised. Post treatment care is easier since there is no large wound or rows of stitches to deal with. The trade off is that the recurrence rate might be higher.

One of the newer techniques being tested is SiLAT (Sinus Laser Therapy). Pappas & Christodoulou (2018) found that using laser energy on a pilonidal sinus could erode the lining, and promote the creation of new healthy tissue as it healed. That new tissue would ideally not lead to the formation of another pilonidal They believe this would be a preferable treatment because it decreases healing time, and is less invasive (Pappas & Christodoulou, 2018). This procedure is still relatively new, and more studies need to be conducted to determine its effectiveness.

Recurrences

The biggest issue with pilonidals is the fact that they can keep coming back again and again even after a successful surgery.

A recurrence can occur months or years down the line and it can feel like it happens for no apparent reason. This can be especially frustrating when we think we are cured and all of a sudden a painful cyst comes screaming back into our lives to make us suffer.

The recurrence rate has been found to range between 20-40% of all patients (Aithal, Rajan & Reddy, 2012). A recurrence after surgery might happen as a result of many different factors. Some of them we can influence, and others are out of our hands.

One of the most crucial factors in recurrences might involve poor wound care after surgery (Yoldas, et al., 2013). When our tissue is repairing and rebuilding itself after an excision there is a lot of activity in the area. Layers upon layers of muscle tissue, and fat are being created and there is plenty of opportunity for another sinus to form. Debris can allow for gaps and tunnels to develop. Infections can damage the tissue. Trauma from sitting or bumping into things can cause internal damage to the tender flesh and again open up the risk of a pilonidal.

After my second pilonidal excision I had stitches down my midline, right between the cheeks, and I was scared of touching them. When I showered I would let soap wash over them, but not do much else. I did not use a shower glove or any other scrub. The flesh was tender and hurt to touch. It was also hard to see what I was doing back there and it seemed wrong to try and get into my crevice to scrub above the stitches. I did not want to do it, and no one at the hosptial gave me any specific instructions to do so.

When I went in for a check up my doctor was upset with me because I didn't scrub right above the stitches, and I had built up some debris. That may have led to the formation of my third pilonidal, which was unfortunate because the fibers of the stitches themselves made it easy for things to get stuck in there.

I now understand that another pilonidal can be brought about by things like a buildup of dead tissue, debris, sweating, and friction in the crevice. Which means that the stitches have to get scrubbed if they are down the midline. Doing it gently is important because we don't want to damage the skin. Even after the wound heals it doesn't mean we are in the clear. We can keep the wound clean, safe, and free from infection but even then as the cleft is rebuilt, a sinus can still find a window of opportunity. It's not always our fault so don't beat yourself up if you think you did everything right with wound care and still developed a recurrence.

Another crucial component affecting the probability of a recurrence is the type of surgery we receive. Stauffer et al. (2018) searched through 740 studies that had been published on pilonidal cyst treatments from 1833 to 2017, and examined the connections between recurrence rates, follow up times, and the surgical procedures utilized. In total there were 80,000 patients over 18 decades included in their research review. They found that Karydakis and Bascom Cleft lift procedures showed the lowest recurrence rates. As I mentioned before, some research has found the recurrence rate for Bascom Cleft to be as low as 8%. Their results also proposed that incision and drainage procedures have a recurrence rate that increases from 25.9% two years after treatment, to 40.2% after 5 years. The findings support the idea that incision and drainage might be less effective at preventing a recurrence (Stauffer et al. 2018).

Here's what I think we can learn from all of this. Getting rid of a pilonidal is only half the battle because afterwards we have to continue working to prevent a recurrence. This is unfortunately one thing that isn't talked about enough by the doctors who treat it. Oftentimes we might see them for one or two post-surgery appointments, but that might involve a visual examination of the wound and not much else.

Doctors can tell us if a wound looks infected, but I haven't heard of many who go into detail regarding preventative measures. For first timers this won't be very helpful because they won't learn about the chances of developing another pilonidal, and many leave their doctors' office thinking the problem has been solved. Hope might lie in a combination of better treatment options and more information for pilonidal sufferers to understand how they can deal with this condition.

I believe that there are very smart people out there who are trying to come up with better ways to treat pilonidals without needing to go through a whole surgery. With advances in technology, I am hopeful that in this decade or the next we can get rid of pilonidals on the first try without having to get a piece of our body cut out. Also, with better access to information I expect that more patients will be able to avoid common mistakes and have an easier time dealing with this condition.

Home Remedies

Surgeries and other medical treatments are not always available to everyone. Some people don't have insurance, can't afford treatment, or don't have any available time for it. Others suffer from a different condition that takes priority over a pilonidal. There are also those that are just too afraid to go see a doctor and want to solve the problem themselves.

Home remedies are usually promoted to fill the need for people in those situations. If you fall into any of those categories or can't seek medical treatment for other reasons, you will probably find online posts and videos that have stuck out to you because they offer possible at-home solutions. Over the years I have read testimonies from those who claim that they successfully treated, or have managed their pilonidal using only herbs, creams, castor oil, tea tree oil, epsom salt baths, or some type of ointment.

The claims are different across the board but it is important to differentiate between curing a pilonidal, and simply managing it with the use of home remedies. Some say that these treatments have stopped their pilonidal from flaring up and they can live a more normal life because they have seen no sign of a recurrence.

Others have used these remedies on swollen and infected pilonidals to make them burst and drain, without getting rid of the pilodial, which is still a win for them because that's what they wanted. They were only looking to get the fluid to release and not much else. These individuals didn't cure their pilonidal they only learned how to manage them.

Regarding the pilonidal sufferers that claim their pilonidal has disappeared, and is gone for good after using home remedies, that is a tough one for me to believe. It might happen in very rare cases, but it's more likely that the remedies have made their pilonidal go dormant. I believe the sinus remains under the skin, but the symptoms and outward visible signs are not present. Home remedies should be done with caution and with an understanding that it might only be the symptoms that are being treated and not the root cause.

Here is an example of a home remedy that might help relieve some of the pain from a pilonidal. If you have a swollen or infected cyst, epsom salt baths are promoted as a way to make it burst and drain. First you fill a bathtub with hot water, enough for it to flow over your cyst as you lay down. It shouldn't be boiling hot because that could burn your skin and you end up in more pain. Then, you add in some epsom salt, which you can find at most pharmacies, and soak in the tub for 15 minutes. This might make your pilonidal come to a head and start draining. After some of the debris and fluid is flushed out you might feel less pain and get some relief.

I tried remedies like this one and others when I was dealing with a painful pilonidal, but I never had any success with them. I have applied tea tree oil and actually felt like it made the situation worse. But, since everyone's pilonidal and body can respond differently to treatments, I can see how some of this stuff would work for others.

In extreme cases I have seen videos and read stories from people who have tried to lance the cyst themselves at home. Out of desperation they used whatever knife or razor they had and cut into the pilonidal to free up the fluid. I have never seen any follow up information months or years later from those who have claimed to be pilonidal free after trying this. This is definitely one thing I would completely avoid because this is a medical condition that requires professional care. For most people, even with the relief they get from home remedies, it will most likely be necessary to have one of the previously discussed surgeries to remove the pilonidal.

If you are not sure whether you are dealing with a pilonidal sinus, or if you're worried that you might be getting hit with another one, and reading all the previous information has raised some concerns for you, I would suggest that you set up an appointment with a doctor and get that figured out right away.

Some of you might feel too embarrassed to talk about it, and you have a lot of anxiety about going to a doctor and pulling down your pants. I wouldn't worry about all of that. Doctors spend their days looking at some pretty messed up stuff and your ass will not be the most memorable thing in their life. Also when it comes to talking to friends, family, or partners about it we might feel like they will judge us, but usually they are only curious. It is much easier to go through this when you feel like you are not alone and can talk to others about the experience so try to open up.

Many people try to self-diagnose, convince themselves that it's harmless, or wait for it to go away on its own. Eventually the realization hits that it can quickly get worse. Random Google searches can lead you down a rabbit hole of home remedies, videos of people lancing their own cyst, and discussions of miracle cures. I won't argue that this stuff hasn't worked for others, but this is a medical issue. One of the best things you can do is get professional treatment to remove it, and then take care of the area to reduce the chance of a recurrence.

There are different treatment options, lifestyle factors, and wound care strategies to take into account, but at the end of the day we are dealing with a huge pain in the ass and we can't ignore the impact it has on our lives. As you will see from my personal stories the cyst can be a confusing thing to figure out on your own. I learned a ton of lessons after every one of my pilonidals, and I am a better person for it today. Everything starts from the very first sign of a pilonidal, and from there on out it is a lifelong journey.

THE FIRST PILONIDAL

The first one was the size of a golf ball. I had recently started college, approaching my 19th birthday, and was going through rapid life changes. I was partying hard almost every weekend and taking on a full-time course load. I was young, energetic, and could easily pull off all nighters. I would show up to class every day after chugging some coffee or energy drinks, and get all my assignments done on time. I felt great and in perfect health.

Before college, I never had any issues with cysts but I do recall one incident where I fell off an ATV right onto my tailbone. I walked it off and was only sore for a few days. Other than that, I had a plump, healthy butt that got me through four years of high school sitting in classrooms all day.

It wasn't until I was fully immersed in college that the trouble started. I remember feeling a small bump right below my tailbone during a workout at the gym. When I saw the bump in a mirror I thought it was an odd place to get a pimple, and completely ignored it. I had started bench pressing and squatting regularly for the first time and believed the exercises were making me breakout in weird places. It was my dumb logic but I truly believed it would die off in a day or two. But the pimple quickly grew bigger.

It wasn't painful and didn't look dangerous, so I kept brushing it off as unimportant. It should have popped and finished its gross existence after a few days, but when it refused to erupt I got frustrated. I locked myself in my bathroom and pressed on it to move the process along. The damn thing wouldn't budge, and that's when I got worried. It started to look big, inflamed, and was becoming painfully sensitive. I forced myself to make a doctors appointment and get it examined.

My primary doctor checked it out and decided it was an infected spider bite. I was relieved to have a diagnosis and left the hospital with some antibiotics that were supposed to kill off the infection within a couple of weeks. I was confident that it would be gone soon and continued with school and working out. As expected the bump grew smaller over the course of two weeks. The pain subsided, and I basically went back to ignoring it.

Eventually I was on the verge of running out of medecine and the bump was still there. Not only that, but it started growing again. I was upset and eagerly waited to see the doctor at the follow up appointment. The days started crawling by. I tried to stay focused on my schoolwork, but during one of my classes fluid began to leak out of it. I sat there as I felt the stream trickle down my butt, terrified that someone might see a bloody stain on my jeans.

I had to leave the room and run to a bathroom where I stuffed toilet paper into my pants to catch all the weird colored blood. In one of the stalls I got a look at my ruined underwear and realized how bad things had gotten. With some paper stuffed into my butt I finished up my day and rushed to leave campus.

I went home that day feeling very scared. My parents, who meant well, recommended that I use their "parche gris", a thick paste with a strong chemical odor, to get rid of it. According to them, it was a remedy from their old Mexican town that they used when something strange appeared on their body. They would smear that weird paste on, and it would suck out all the bad stuff. I decided it couldn't hurt to try since the antibiotics were all but gone at that point. I smeared the paste over the bump and covered it with a large band-aid.

A few hours later I had to use the bathroom. While sitting down on the toilet I felt liquid falling from my butt again. I looked into the bowl and saw drops of blood, followed by a whole stream of it. I freaked out. My parent's remedy had worked, but a little too well. *I'm going to bleed to death!* I thought. In a panic I got naked and washed the paste off in the shower.

After seeing all that blood I thought the bump would be gone for sure. I dried myself and examined my backside in the bathroom mirror. The damn thing was still there. The miracle remedy had failed. *Now it looks like a volcano,* I thought. And that was the end of that experiment. The top of it had come to a point almost like a little missle wanted to shoot out of it.

My follow up appointment arrived and I updated the doctor on everything that had taken place. She decided that it was time to see a specialist because the thing was definitely not an infected spider bite. She had an idea of what it might be, and referred me to a colon and rectal surgeon. That appointment wouldn't arrive for another week, and the thing was starting to get angry.

I sat in my classes wincing in pain whenever it touched the back of my chair, or when my pants brushed against it. I started wearing band-aids throughout the day to capture the blood and fluids that kept leaking out. It continuously drained, and I had to change bandaids in my school's bathroom just to avoid stains through my clothing.

I was also very embarrassed. Terrified that someone might notice I was walking and sitting with an exaggerated posture. I didn't want to tell anyone what was going on, and I would lie when someone would ask me about my strange behavior. It was turning into a very depressing time. My only option was to suck it up until I could finally see the specialist.

After a brutal week, I went in to see the colon and rectal surgeon. Unlike other hospital rooms he had his own office space with two nurses and nothing more. I awkwardly sat in the waiting room chair with only one butt cheek on it. It was getting too painful to sit properly. When my turn came up I walked into the examination room where the doctor was waiting.

He was a middle aged man with a serious face and calm demeanor. As I explained my symptoms, he was already putting on gloves. Before I finished speaking, he told me to pull down my pants and lay face down on the hospital bed. I did as instructed and showed him the bump. I prayed that he wouldn't touch it but of course that's the first thing he did. Within a few seconds, and some quick painful presses on the area, he confirmed that I had an infected pilonidal cyst and I would need to have surgery to remove it.

I froze and repeated his words in my head because that didn't sound right. I tried to question him and make him realize that he was making a mistake.

"Are you sure?" I asked. "My primary doctor mentioned a spider bite, could it be that?"

As he removed the gloves and washed his hands, he explained everything very clearly.

"This needs to be surgically removed or it will burrow down to your spine, and could lead to much bigger problems for you."

I was shocked. *Burrow down to your spine,* his words echoed in my head. *I've never had a surgery before, oh my God this is horrible.* It destroyed me to hear that such a small insignificant thing was forcing me under the knife.

"Does your family have any history with cysts?" He asked, breaking my train of thought.

"No, they haven't had anything like this," I answered.

"Is your family from any Mediterranean countries?" He continued.

"Not that I know of."

"I ask because I usually see this in patients with a lot of thick, coarse hair from Mediterranean regions," he said, and with that, the questions ended.

He grabbed his appointment book and we set a date for

the operation right there on the spot. I went with the motions, pretending to check my availability, but I wasn't all there. I was losing it. To top it all off the earliest available slot was the morning before Thanksgiving. I left the office with fear building up inside me, and immediately started researching pilonidal cyst when I got home.

I needed to know everything about it. The tons of images and videos I found intensified my nervous energy. As I kept learning more about the condition, I realized this was going to leave me bedridden for a while. I took a medical leave from school, and cancelled my Thanksgiving plans. It looked like I would be spending my holiday secretly recovering. I didn't want to tell any of my friends what was about to happen. I was too embarrassed, and felt it was shameful to have an operation around my ass.

I also had to blow off a date with a nice girl to avoid telling her about my situation. I met up with her right after a morning class to explain everything and basically lied.

"I can't go out with you like we planned," I told her. "I'm going to Mexico to visit my family for Thanksgiving, but I will let you know when I get back."

I said it in a hurried manner, trying to get it over with quickly. She looked very surprised.

"When will you be back?" She asked.

"I'm not sure," I said.

It hurt to lie.

"Why don't you know when you'll come back?"

"I figure I'll come back when I'm ready, and I don't know when I will be ready just yet."

It was an odd answer and I left it at that. She could tell that I was being closed off and didn't push any further.

My life came to a complete stop, and I prepared for the worst. Time passed slowly and I could barely take a step without feeling a shot of pain from the cyst. It was a constant reminder that I was soon going to have a piece of my body cut out.

The night before the surgery was very frustrating. I wasn't allowed to eat or drink anything, other than water, about 8-10 hours before the operation. Since I had to arrive to the hospital by 8am, I stopped eating around 9pm. I showered with a special soap provided by the surgeon's office to clean germs and bacteria off my body. It was hard to get it to lather and I scrubbed for a long time trying to remove all the germs from my skin.

I went to bed by 10pm, but it was hard to sleep. I tossed and turned rolling from my side to my stomach, avoiding any pressure on the cyst. I had been getting a sore back from not being able to lay down comfortably, and it made that night all the more uncomfortable. You can bet I was still googling things for hours and watching videos on pilonidals. I finally dozed off around midnight with the cyst pulsating and negative thoughts running through my head.

The next morning I was eager to get going as soon as I woke up. A twinge of pain from the cyst had become a regular greeting when I got out of bed. This time was no different. It let me know it was still there and wasn't going away without a fight. I was hungry, anxious, scared, and very sleepy. More than anything I wanted it out of my body fast and rushed to get ready.

As my mom drove me to the hospital, my mind was firmly focused on surviving. We sat quietly the whole way in her beaten down van. It was a gloomy day and rain was expected. The weather definitely fit my general vibe. All over the city, people were waking up to make preparations for Thanksgiving. There was a festive atmosphere, even with the poor weather, and it made me feel lonelier. *I am on my way to have a piece of my body cut out!* I screamed in my head. The fear was nauseating.

We arrived at the hospital. I walked in through the sliding doors, and straight to the front desk where I was greeted by an older lady. She typed away at the computer, confirmed my appointment, then directed me to a waiting room after I filled out some quick paperwork. It was early morning and surprisingly empty for such a large hospital. I figured the doctor would be at his best if I was the first one to be operated on. Then I thought he might also be sleepy and mess up. I was freaking myself out and had to snap out of it, but it's hard to not think about the worst while sitting inside a hospital.

I sat quietly watching the news on an outdated TV, while my mom browsed through some magazines. After 15 minutes my nurse, a middle aged woman with tired eyes, walked in and called my name. She immediately led us down some winding hallways, making small talk along the way.

We arrived at a room with enough space for two beds, a table, and some chairs. An old man was already lying down on the first bed closest to the door and bathroom. He was accompanied by, who I assumed was, his wife. She was sitting next to him and smiled at us as we entered. The old man was not in a smiling mood and I didn't blame him. I was right there with him on that one. I walked over to my bed next to a large window with a view of the thick fog outside, and awkwardly stood next to it.

The nurse brought over a hospital gown, some socks, and a bag. Her instructions were clear. I had to take off all my clothes, put on the hospital garments, and lay down on the bed. She drew a sliding curtain all around the bed to give me some privacy. I changed while my mom waited on the other side of my makeshift cocoon.

I put my clothes into the plastic bag and tied up the gown before climbing onto the bed. I had to lay on my back. As soon as I settled in, the cyst hit me with another burst of pain. I could feel it all the way up to my head and I clenched my teeth. The curtains were pulled aside, and my mom took a seat in a chair next to me.

We both watched as the nurse began prepping some equipment on a small table. First, she put an ID tag on my wrist with my general information. Then, she got started on the IV. There was a needle at one end, with a small container, and a long narrow tube attached to it. The tube led all the way up to a bag that was half full with a clear liquid. The bag was hanging from a tall pole.

I caught a glimpse of the needle and turned away. I felt very vulnerable lying there naked under a gown, while the nurse prepared to inject me. I heard her shuffle an inch closer and I braced myself. She grabbed my arm, told me to make a tight fist and then relax it. The needle was pushed into the top of my hand right between my knuckles and wrist. A quick pinch and it was done. Not as bad as I expected. She fastened the needle to my hand with some tape and moved on to the next task.

I took some quick breaths and looked over at my hand. There it was, my first IV. The needle was beneath my skin with a small tube attached to it on the outside. The tape kept the needle securely strapped down, but I didn't feel confident moving my hand. The attached tube snaked its way up to the IV bag that was now hanging off the metal pole which was moved above my head.

I was starting to get freaked out by everything and my mom probably noticed. She reassured me that the needle wouldn't slip out or hurt me if I moved. I was almost 19 and still needed my mom to comfort me. The nurse joined in and said, "It's ok, let me know if it bothers you." After a minute I moved my hand carefully and it felt fine.

The nurse started gathering her things, gave me the remote to another outdated TV, and left the room. An hour had now passed since arriving at the hospital. I laid on the bed and wondered what was coming next.

Time was moving slowly, and outside the gloomy day had turned into pouring rain. *Crazy weather,* I thought. I was worried that it would somehow impact the surgeon's performance. Maybe the lights will go out, or a thunderstorm could hit and break his concentration. The worst case scenarios raced through my mind.

The nurse returned after a few minutes to check in on me, and explained that the anesthesiologist would be dropping by to discuss the procedure. This was the person in charge of putting me to sleep, making sure I didn't wake up mid-operation, and that I came back after it was all over.

The anesthesiologist walked in. A kind looking little lady with a gentle smile. She explained how I would be put to sleep, and asked some general questions about my medical history. I then asked what I felt were important questions.

"Is there any chance I wake up mid-surgery?" "How long will I be out?" "Will I know I am being put to sleep as it happens?" "Will it hurt?"

All her answers were concise.

"Everything will be fine," she said confidently. "I will make sure you don't wake up. It will take a few hours depending on the size of the cyst. You will be asleep before you realize it, and it will not hurt."

After this quick talk she headed out to get ready for the surgery.

An hour and a half after arriving to the hospital, it was almost time. The nurse came back to make it official.

She moved the curtains out of the way and said, "Ok, let's get you in there, say bye to momma!"

I glanced over at my mom who looked back at me with wide eyes. She hugged me, said a prayer, and tried to convince me everything was going to be okay.

"There's nothing to worry about," she said.

But I could see her holding back tears. The nurse pushed on

the bed and released the wheel locks. I started rolling out of the room right past the old man and his visitor. In a strange way the ride to the operation room was actually fun. I was gliding down some long hallways and got to see the hustle and bustle of the facility. I caught glimpses of different patients in their rooms and wondered if they were all going through a similar experience. Unfortunately, the ride didn't last long. I wished it would have.

The nurse pushed me past some swinging doors, down a very short hallway, and into the surgery room. There was an immediate drop in the temperature. I shivered under my gown. The room held about six strangers all in full surgical gear with gloves, face masks, and caps on their heads. If my surgeon was in there I wouldn't know it.

Everyone was busy preparing with their backs to me. When they turned around only their eyes were visible. The room held all types of equipment. Large, bright lights illuminated a single bed in the middle of the room. I avoided looking at all the metal tables holding the tools that I believed would be used to cut into me.

I was wheeled in and the bed came to a stop. I was asked to get up and shuffle onto the other surgery bed. I stood up and awkwardly waddled over. The nurse helped move the IV bag along with me. As I transitioned, I was actually nervous about someone seeing through the huge opening in the back of my gown. They were all going to be looking at my ass for a few hours, but I still felt embarrassed. As I laid down, the cyst shot out a final painful bolt. *Get this damn thing out of me!* I screamed in my head, as the lights above beamed down on me.

I looked around and my nurse was already out of the room. I

didn't even realize it. She took my bed on wheels with her and the doors were shut. There was no turning back now.

Two strangers immediately started taping things to my body, I assumed to measure my vitals. A third person joined them and I noticed it was the anesthesiologist by the look of her eyes. She placed an oxygen mask over my mouth and nose, and instructed me to take deep breaths. I inhaled. The air was cool and clean. It felt good as it entered my lungs. I exhaled, and felt like Darth Vader.

It seemed like everyone in the room had moved closer to me. I was wondering when the anesthesia was going to start working, and within four or five breaths I was out. It felt like my eyes were open one second, and the next there was only darkness and silence.

Suddenly I heard sounds in the distance. I had no idea where I was or what was happening. I only knew that I was very tired and wanted to keep my eyes closed. My mind had other plans as it slowly brought me back into consciousness. I was surrounded by pitch blackness, and the sounds around me were pulling me out of it. I tried opening my eyes, but they wouldn't respond. I felt too exhausted and wanted nothing more than to sleep.

At the same time, I couldn't keep myself from waking up. The noises around me grew clearer, I cracked my eyelids open, and saw a blurry figure by my feet.

The nurse greeted me, "Welcome back."

As I shuffled my head I tried keeping my eyes open, but I was stuck in a limbo between sleeping and waking up. An unknown amount of time later I was able to speak.

In a raspy tone I asked, "What happened?"

The nurse quickly answered, "Everything went well, and you are all done. The surgery was a success. The doctor removed the cyst. It was large and deep. He said it was about the size of a golf ball. That means the wound will probably be big too."

I didn't know if I should have felt scared, or relieved that it was done. Minute by minute I regained control of my body and feeling in my face.

My lips were dry, I was thirsty, and my throat hurt. The nurse had water ready for me. Once I was able to sip on it she brought in my mom who looked as exhausted as I felt. It took about 40 minutes before I was fully awake and alert. I felt mounds of bandages along my butt, but no pain. The nurse removed all the cords and clamps attached to me and let me know that I was free to go once I used the bathroom. They wanted to make sure my body was functioning internally before I headed out.

She gave me instructions for open wound care and some supplies to take with me for gauze changes. I went to the bathroom after about one hour. Then I changed into my regular clothes with my mom's help. Out of fear I didn't dare bend over too much. My bones felt heavy and stiff.

I walked out of the hospital with small baby steps. I was offered a wheelchair, but declined. I was worried about sitting down after the surgery and didn't want to risk any tearing. I wasn't sure how an open wound worked, but I treated it with extreme caution. I slowly shuffled towards the front entrance while my mom brought the van over from the parking lot.

Instead of getting into the passenger seat I laid down in the back. I was too scared to sit. I must have looked ridiculous lying on my belly as my mom shut the door behind me but I didn't care. We got home and I shuffled into the house. My dad greeted me at the door.

"How did it go?" He looked very serious as always.

I didn't answer. I was feeling very grumpy and tired at that point. I immediately walked to my bed and slid myself on to it. I let some movies play in the background and the rest of the day passed in a haze until I fell asleep on my side.

I woke up groggy and anxious the following morning. It was officially time for my first shower and to change all the gauze that was packed into the wound. I tried to stall by eating breakfast and watching TV, but it was inevitable. The hospital gave us a number for an in-home nursing agency. We were told to call and set up some recurring appointments for gauze changes. The person we scheduled to do wound care at our house was not arriving until late in the afternoon, which meant the first gauze change had to be done without the extra help and my mom would be packing in the new gauze. She was as nervous as I was.

I walked into the bathroom, closed the door, and took a long look at myself in our large mirror. I turned around. The mirror was barely long enough for me to see the medical tape and bandages covering the top half of my butt. It looked like a small diaper. I started peeling everything away slowly. I was terrified of what I was going to see or even damaging the wound if I moved too quickly. The minutes dragged on, and I started to sweat.

The first layer of tape and bandages came off like a small pad. There was more gauze underneath. I could see dried blood and knew I was getting close. The second layer had no tape to hold it in place and came off easily. Once off it revealed the gauze that was packed inside the wound. Beneath this third layer, I would see the size and depth of the damage. It was difficult to grip since it was tightly packed around the wound. I tugged and felt a slight resistance.

It freaked me out. *What was I pulling at? Was it stuck to my wound? What if it started to hurt? Am I supposed to just suck it up and deal with it? I should have taken painkillers!* I thought. I pinched and pulled on the gauze and felt it edge out a little. *Okay,* I thought, *progress!* Next came a moderately harder tug. The gauze stretched out and unfolded slowly. A square piece finally let loose, and I was that much closer to the finish line.

The trash can was filling up with the bandages. I took some shallow breaths and moved on to the next clump that was sticking out from the wound. I could see the edges of the wound and more gauze packed snuggly inside it. The wound had the shape of a triangle. This is where things got tougher. Every touch in the area made me flinch. I can't say that any of this hurt, only felt unnatural. After some frustrating seconds and with full streams of sweat falling down my forehead, I was able to get enough of the gauze between my fingers to start pulling.

It felt attached to the inside of the wound. The dried blood and fluids causing an adhesive effect. I shuttered as I tugged. The stubborn thing wouldn't budge. I gave myself some motivational words. *Suck it up and pull you punk!* I thought. "It's not that easy!" I yelled back at myself, out loud. It was becoming a 30-minute ordeal.

I paused, looked myself in the eyes and asked, "Would you rather have the cyst back?" The answer was easy. I pinched at the gauze, caught a good grip, and pulled with steady force, then a bit harder, and a bit harder. I didn't let up to regrip or rest. My hand was shaking, but the gauze slid out of the hole a few centimeters. Oh, what a sweet feeling it was. I could now see the gauze was shaped like a shoelace instead of a square chunk. It was going to be one long piece. I took a moment to analyze it and went back to pulling.

The gauze started sliding out. Inch by inch it came out, every so often getting stuck, but with some cautious yanking, it continued moving. I now had a 12-inch tail coming out of the wound and had to regrip closer to the hole. The inside of the wound was taking shape, how deep it went I was still not sure. The tugging continued. With the last piece holding on stubbornly, I tore it out with some frustration. There it was, my triangle shaped gaping wound.

It was strange seeing the inside of my body for the first time. The wound scared me, but at least I knew what I was working with. It was located on the inner edge of my right butt cheek. I could see the meat and inner workings of my ass. It was hard not to stare for a while.

I was able to shower without much issue and, as instructed, I made sure to let water rinse out the wound. I took the detachable shower head and sprayed hot water straight into the wound. I finished up, dried off, and went to lie down on my bed. I didn't even want my towel to touch the wound so I walked half naked to my bed.

It was time for my mom to pack the wound with new gauze. We were both nervous. I gripped my pillow tight and shoved my face into it. We had bought the long shoelace type gauze and some saline to moisten it up. My mom took the gauze and with a cuetip started pushing it into the wound. I felt it going in and kept telling her to be careful. She was being extremely cautious, but I couldn't help myself.

I needed to keep repeating out loud, "Be careful, be careful!"

I felt the gauze reach the bottom of the wound.

"I am being careful," she said as she concentrated.

She was using the cue tip to guide the long lace of gauze in and pressing ever so slightly to make sure it was filling in the wound. An unnatural, uncomfortable sensation was flowing from the area. It was not pleasant, and I bit into my pillow to keep from yelling. My mom finished up, covered the wound with a few square pieces of gauze, and secured it with medical tape. I laid there afterwards and took slow, deep breaths. It was done, but I would have to do this over and over again.

My days now consisted of changing the gauze in the morning and afternoon, and trying not to move too much. The in-home nurse became a regular visitor who helped make the process easier. I was terrified of bending over, using the bathroom, or even getting into bed and laying on my back. I ate standing up, slept on my stomach, and shuffled around very slowly everywhere I went.

Most of this experience involved overcoming a mental block of fear.

One of the scariest parts was using the toilet. I actually tried to hold off on going for as long as I could, but my body needed to do its business. To make the first time easier I held up my body weight with the sink's countertop. I didn't want to squat and actually tried going while laying down backwards over the toilet, but the mechanics were all off. I had to slightly bend my body, as little as possible in order to start pushing, and tried to get it over with. My arm strength eventually gave out and I ended up sitting all the way down, but I wouldn't dare get comfortable. It was a few days before I used it normally.

I also had to get used to the gauze changes. Having to pull it out and have someone push new gauze in was an invasive sensation. We had about three different nurses showing up to the house in rotations to do the wound care. One guy in particular was much rougher and always in a hurry. That wasn't fun. The only benefit was that he got it over with much faster, like ripping off a band-aid. Except the band-aid is being shoved into the wound in this scenario.

Eventually, the hole started closing up and we ran out of in-home nurse appointments. It was up to my parents again. They were fast learners and did a great job. As the entrance to the wound healed, they needed to use the cue tip to make sure they reached the bottom of the miniature cave. I was given painkillers to make this whole thing easier, but I was concerned about getting addicted, and overall I didn't really need them.

Sometimes there would be a pinch of pain, but mostly it was

general discomfort that came with the sensations of wound care. My dad was definitely a bit clumsier, and it wasn't fun having him start pushing in the gauze only to realize he forgot the cue tip or his glasses. This happened a few times and I started carrying his glasses around when it was time to have the gauze changed.

This wound took about 1 month to close up. However, I was able to sit normally and do regular activities within 2 weeks of the operation. When the time came to return to normal life, I did it with the expectation that I would never have to deal with this again. I was happy and had a lot of catching up to do with my friends and school work. I thought everything would be great from that point on. I went back to my regular routine and forgot all about it. I thought the first pilonidal was going to be a random event in my life that would be nothing more than an interesting story to tell, but I was wrong.

THE DEPRESSING
PILONIDAL

I knew it had returned immediately. Month's after my first operation I still remembered the feeling well, but I foolishly thought it was a thing of the past. I was happy until this pilonidal pulled me back into pure sadness.

It was a nice weekend and I was on a date with a girl I had met in school. We were walking into a restaurant for dinner before heading out to a movie. Absolutely nothing was wrong up to that point. We sat down at a booth, and as I pushed back to settle into my seat, I felt a sharp pressure below my tailbone that shot up my spine all the way up to my throat. *It's back!* I thought.

I paused for a second. Maybe I am just imagining it. Maybe it's the scar from the previous surgery acting up. While my date settled in and flipped through the menu I forced myself to press my butt into the seat and confirm what I already knew to be true. I felt it again. I turned red hot and uneasy. My date hadn't noticed. The waiter walked over and asked us if we wanted anything to drink to start off. I was getting lost in my thoughts. *It's back, the bastard is back!*

I looked blankly ahead until my date asked, "Are you okay?"

"Yea," I said. "It's just warm in here..."

I called this one the depressing pilonidal. This reincarnation sucked me back into the turmoil. With my first surgery behind me I thought I was in the clear. I had taken it easy and let my body heal. I was glad to have survived the procedure and went on with my life, intent on forgetting all about it. I wondered what I could have done differently.

Throughout the course of that date, the pressure worsened. As we ate our food I had to start arching my back to avoid making contact with my seat. I tried to stay calm as I talked with my date, but I wondered to myself, *should I tell her? It would be nice to get it all out. But, what if she's grossed out by it?* I couldn't risk it. I didn't say anything about it, and we went on to a movie after eating.

I sat in that theater adjusting myself the entire time unable to get comfortable. When it was over, I rushed to end the date and go home to examine myself. I drove my date to her house quickly, and gave her a fast goodbye. I couldn't think clearly and the conversation had gone no where the whole evening. I was pretty sure I had blown it, or as I thought then, the pilonidal blew it for me.

I got home, looked in the bathroom mirror, and saw the tiniest bump in the exact location of the previous cyst. I was in deep denial and refused to believe what I was seeing. I went to bed and completely avoided lying on my back. *Maybe I only need to let my butt rest and everything will be okay tomorrow,* I thought.

When I touched the area the next day I surprisingly felt no pain and convinced myself that it must be the scar adjusting itself. I went about my week with a constant focus on the area, searching for the slightest discomfort. I felt nothing, and wondered if I exaggerated the sensations during the date. I wanted to be sure and scheduled an appointment with the surgeon who had operated on me. I prayed he would tell me I was being paranoid.

I was able to see him the following week and by the time I went in, the discomfort had begun to increase again. It was on and off, not a consistent pain like the previous pilonidal.

The surgeon recognized me when I walked into his office and quickly asked, "Is it bothering you again?"

"It is, but I think it might just be the scar," I replied.

He took a look, pressed on the area, and confirmed that the cyst was back. It hurt to hear that. I cried inside and felt the energy drain from my body. I tried to be positive.

"Luckily I caught it early and it's going to be a much smaller excision, right? I asked him.

"We won't know until we get in there," he answered.

That was not reassuring. Last time it ended up being the size of a golf ball, and I didn't find that out until I was recovering from the anesthesia.

I tried to remain positive as the days rolled by before heading back to the surgery room again, but the positivity turned into pure sadness. I was less afraid this time, but much more miserable. I kept asking why this was happening to me and drowning in self pity.

I had to cancel plans in preparation for post-operation recovery, and disappeared again into exile. I suffered alone and filled myself with negativity. I again started to obsessively scan through web pages and articles that discussed pilonidal cyst. Nothing I came across gave me any relief. I was consuming much of the same information as the previous time, but it was as if I was reading it all for the first time.

During one depressing session of random Google searches, I came across a support group and was amazed at how many stories were being shared by people experiencing the same turmoil. These forums became a great space to vent my frustration and meet other people with pilonidal cyst. The loneliness faded when I discovered the millions of people suffering through this and I was filled up with hope.

I wasn't going into this alone, I was part of a large collection of people struggling to overcome it. The forums connected me with new insights and inspirational messages. They helped me enormously through a very difficult time. I stayed connected to those support groups until the day of my surgery.

I went in for the operation, and everything went well. It all followed the same process. I was put to sleep and brought back after it was over. I laid on that hospital bed with my sore throat, dry lips, and wondered if it would be the last time.

I was sent home after recovering from the anesthesia with the same instructions to shower the following day and change the gauze. I had some DVD's ready to go and spent the first day back watching movies. I was nauseous and felt very sleepy, but the feeling was now more familiar.

The next day I checked on the wound and got myself ready to start doing the wound changes. I looked in the mirror, had the trash can set up, and was surprised to find that the wound was completely closed up. There was no gauze to pull out. All I saw was a row of stitches gripping a raw, bloody scar, right from the top of my butt crack down to my butthole. There was nothing else.

It turned out the doctor had done a closed wound excision. I did not have to worry about packing it with gauze and it was much easier to deal with. The area was sore and felt tight, but it didn't bother me beyond that. All I had to do was tape a square layer of gauze over it, and be very careful as I went about my day.

My biggest fear was tearing it open. I didn't want to bend over or use the toilet because I thought the stitches would break and I would end up in the emergency room. This kept me on high alert but those fears quickly faded.

I got comfortable with the closed wound, returned to school within a week, and sat in all my classes. I was very cautious, but by the end of that first school day, I realized I may have gone back too soon, and decided to take a few more days off. It felt like strings were tightening around it and I did not like that.

After a restful weekend I was back in school and only felt the occasional twinge of pain. Within a week and a half the thin wound appeared to be completely healed and there was only a tender scar. I went to a follow up appointment with my surgeon who checked on my progress after two weeks. He looked at the stitches nestled within the cleft of my butt as I laid face down.

After a pause he started scolding me for not scrubbing the area better to keep it clean. I was surprised to hear that. I thought I was supposed to avoid messing with the stitches. He showed me some of the debris that had built up, and I reassured him that I would start scrubbing right on the scar. According to him I needed to make sure and reach into the cleft of my butt even if it hurt to touch. This would have been great to know before I got the stitches, but the only instructions I ever got where to shower the day after surgery.

The stitches were still poking through my skin and I asked if they were going to be removed. He said it was not necessary, but offered to take them out. I felt the sutures slide out of my skin and it hurt a lot more than I expected. The strong, painful pinch continued until they all came out. I left the office with a sore butt, a huge smile, and again feeling very relieved to be all done with pilonidals.

Since I spent a lot of time sitting while playing computer games and working on assignments, I decided to buy a coccyx cushion to take pressure off my tailbone and used it for a while. I even worked on my poor posture and started to sit up straight. At the time I was motivated by the fear of another pilonidal.

Within a month of recovering, I stopped using the cushion when sitting, and forgot about my posture. I also stopped visiting the online forums and support groups, and no longer felt like I needed to be a part of the community. When I was able to get through a gym session without any discomfort, I took it as a sign that I was back to one-hundred percent.

I forgot the hard lesson I had just learned again, and went back to business as usual. I bounced back from my depression quickly because I had such a fast post-operation recovery. I did not take care of myself and went back to partying and having adventures with friends as if nothing had happened. I should have been more careful, but I wanted to move on with my life and didn't want to think about the depressing pilonidal.

This inevitably impacted me down the road. The wound looked to be healed from the outside, but what I didn't realize was that internally the flesh was still tender. It wasn't until I received an ashiatsu massage, about 1 year later, that I was concerned about a recurrence.

I distinctly remember the masseuse getting up on the table, and then, standing on top of my calves. Apparently, with this style of massage they literally walk on top of you. I didn't ask for it, but figured it would be interesting to try it out, and didn't ask her to stop. She slowly walked up my body while holding on to beams on the roof for balance. She moved up towards my ass, stepped on my left buttcheck then on the right one. With all her weight on top of me, I felt a tiny pop near the cleft of my butt. Other than the weight of someone standing on me, I didn't feel any pain and wondered if that pop had something to do with the scar.

I drove home and kept thinking about the popping sensation. It slipped from my mind after a few hours of not feeling anything, and I didn't think about it again. Maybe I should have called my doctor or gone in for a checkup, but at that time my mind told me, *Don't worry about it, it's nothing. You are fine. There is no way it can come back for a third time.* Everything led me to the same conclusion, ignore it.

I did exactly that and nothing happened the next day, weeks, and months later. Time passed and I would occasionally check myself in the bathroom mirror, but there was nothing out of the ordinary to see. I felt great. *I must be in the clear now,* I reassured myself. *There is no way that I am one of those people that can get this three times. I can't be one of those unlucky people.*

THE SHOCKING
PILONIDAL

T he sheer amount of flesh that was cut out of me left me absolutely shocked. It looked like an extra large ice cream scoop was used on the inside of both my butt cheeks. I thought it would be impossible for my body to heal from this one, and I would be left with a moon size crater on half my ass. This was the shocking pilonidal.

The cyst came back almost a year and a half after the second operation. At this point I had become very frustrated with my two unsuccessful excisions and was looking to try something different. I found some home remedies online and figured it couldn't hurt to give them a shot. I added turmeric to my diet, applied warm compress daily, took epsom salt baths, and used different creams with a variety of ingredients. None of it worked.

The cyst was small, and now it was surrounded by a small scar. My ass had clearly been through some stuff and it looked like I had no choice but to go in for another surgery. I decided that the root of the problem must have been with my surgeon. I ignored the fact that I was living an active lifestyle and treating my butt very poorly. I didn't even take into account the brutal massage I had received.

Instead I focused on finding a new surgeon. I searched through different specialists in the area and came upon one who was receiving good reviews. I made an appointment and went in for a consultation. I should have backed out of this decision as soon as I visited his office.

The waiting room was crammed full of people, and it was messy. I had to wait in the hallway since they were beyond capacity inside the room. After about half an hour the nurse came out to get me, and rushed me into his examination room where I was greeted by a tiny old man. He seemed very erratic.

As I explain my situation he immediately brushed off all my concerns with quick reassuring statements. He was very confident in himself, and claimed that he could get rid of the cyst for good. It would be no big deal for him.

I told him about my issue with two previous surgeries and he said, "Don't worry, I'm going to get it all out. I'm not like other surgeons that do nothing. I will get all of it, and you won't have to worry about it anymore."

That's what I wanted to hear. But I also wanted to mention a procedure I had read about online and see if he could help explain it to me.

"I read about something called a Bascom cleft lift while doing some research. Is that something that we can try?"

"Oh, did you hear?," he said to the nurse who was within earshot in the adjoining room. "He has been doing some research. Good job Alex."

"That's good," the nurse added.

"Thanks..." I replied, unsure if they were being condescending. I didn't know what to say next.

He didn't answer my question, and started listing some available dates for the surgery. We scheduled it, and with that, he sent me on my way. I analyzed what had taken place while driving home. Something didn't feel right, but I was desperate for a solution. I ignored my gut and hoped that this time the procedure was going to work. *It seemed like he knew how pilonidals worked and if the Bascom Cleft Lift was a good technique he would of told me right?* I asked myself. *He's the doctor and he knows what he is doing,* I replied reassuringly.

The excision surgery followed the same process as the previous times, except this hospital was much busier. Everything felt rushed from the moment I arrived with my mom. The nurse attending to me seemed unconcerned with providing a personal touch, and was all about business. My mom was there to support me, but her commentary on the chaos in the hospital made me more nervous.

My anxiety levels peaked that day when I was all prepped for the operation and then left in a hallway, lying on my hospital bed, as I was being wheeled over to the surgery room. Apparently, the room wasn't ready at the time the nurse brought me over, and she had to keep me outside the entry doors for a few minutes. My mom had already said goodbye to me and here I was in a hallway feeling completely alone.

As I laid there on the bed, staring at the ceiling, I regretted my decision to switch doctors. But it was too late to back out now. I was naked under my hospital gown with an IV inserted into me. It was either I do it, or bail and try to get a surgery somewhere else which could take weeks. I didn't want another day with the cyst and stayed on the bed.

When I was finally pushed into the surgery room the anesthesiologist quickly got to work putting me to sleep. There was no oxygen mask this time. Instead, anesthesia was put into me through an IV. I clearly remember the feeling of the cold fluid pushing up through my left arm and past my shoulder. As it reached my head, a sharp, electric pain ran across my face. I began to drift out of consciousness and at the last second muttered, "My face hurts." I don't know if any of them heard me, or if my words were even comprehensible. It's possible they ignored me and went on with the procedure.

In the next instant I was coming out of a deep sleep with a shock. I heard my name being called and tried to gain some bearing. Everything was darkness and I couldn't find my center. The distant echoes of my name grew louder, closer, and clearer. I realized that I was surrounded by a few people trying to wake me up. A tube slid out from deep in my throat and I started coughing. Fluid started filling up the inside of my mouth and going down into my throat. Another tube was quickly shoved in to start sucking up the fluid. I tried not to choke on it and struggled to move.

"Come on buddy…come on," someone said.

What are they talking about? Who are they? I wondered.

I was coming out of the black and into chaos. I started to remember.

Didn't I just close my eyes a few seconds ago? I was in a surgery… Oh that's right, I just had a surgery! When I realized I was coming out of anesthesia, I tried forcing my body to move. I wanted the tube out of my mouth. My eyes were cracking open, but nothing was visible. I wanted to cough and strained to turn my head.

Somebody started massaging my chest and saying, "It's okay, calm down, you're okay."

My body wouldn't respond and I could only shake my legs and vibrate my arms. I had no idea how many people were around me. I forced my eyes to open wider and I could only see two blurry figures on either side of me. I was lying on a bed and continuing to cough up a thick fluid. One person kept working the suction tube in my mouth and the other cleaned up my face.

This isn't normal, this isn't how I wake up from anesthesia, I thought.

"He's coming out," another voice said.

Even in my disoriented state, I knew something was wrong. My throat continued to hurt and I couldn't stop coughing. My strength was returning and I kept reaching for the suction tube.

One of the blurry figures moved my hand off it and tried to calm me down. "You're okay, you're fine, everything is fine."

It doesn't feel fine! I wanted to panic.

After several minutes my eyes were wide open, and I had regained feeling in my arms and legs. Only one nurse was left at my side. The blood was still trickling in throat. She helped me sit up on the bed and let me hold the suction tube. I looked at the fluid flowing through the tube, it was pure dark blood. It was gushing from a cut inside my throat caused by the thing they jerked out of me when I was waking up. I struggled to speak without coughing but could only grumble.

"You had us worried for a bit there," a second nurse said as she walked in, with my mom looking mortified.

"Waah..," I gurgled out.

My mom's face freaked me out and I was sure that something had gone wrong.

"What happened?" My mom asked for me.

The nurse explained that I had difficulty waking up from the anesthesia. The tube that cut me was pumping oxygen into my lungs while they tried to wake me up - my mom was on the verge of tears. I went back to coughing up blood and feeling like crap.

When the bleeding finally stopped and my strength returned, my nurse began to give me the usual post-operation instructions. In that moment I had to use the restroom and simply got up and walked over to the nearby toilet. I tried to listen to hear, but I was so nauseous that I kept walking to the bathroom without letting her finish. I closed the door behind me and started to throw up. Bloody liquid came out of me each time.

The nurse patiently waited next to my mom for me to walk back to the bed before continuing with the instructions. In the end I walked back and forth from the nurse to the bathroom, and threw up three times before she finished talking. Then she sent me on my way. They didn't connect me with an in-home nurse for wound care, but I didn't care. I was too frustrated with the entire ordeal and only wanted to leave.

I coughed up blood all the way home and couldn't get rid of the nauseating feeling. I went right to bed and collapsed for a rough night of sleep. The next day I woke up thinking it was going to be business as usual. Since we had no in-home nurse coming, the gauze changes would have to be done by my parents, but I believed they had practiced enough times to do it with ease. No one at the hospital had told me about the size of the excision which made me think the huge mounds of gauze were a bit unusual. I expected the open wound to be similar in size to the first one.

I went into the bathroom to remove the bandages and see the depth and size of it. I got the trash can ready to drop in the gauze, and made sure to have some paper towels handy. I started with the outer layer of tape and dressings, peeling it off like a huge band aid. Underneath I saw a massive amount of bloody gauze. It looked messier than usual. I grabbed another piece of the padding. It was very closely stuck to my skin. I figured the dried blood was making it cling to my body and there would be more layers underneath. I pulled off this large clump of gauze and my jaw dropped. I completely froze.

I was standing naked, looking over my shoulder at the

mirror and what I saw was horrific. The mound of gauze was not covering up the wound, it was inside the wound! I was removing the packing inside of what turned out to be the biggest wound I had ever seen in my life. The remaining gauze easily fell out and I looked into a cavernous opening. It was as if the surgeon had scooped out the inside of both my butt-cheeks and simply took out pounds of flesh and meat. There was no precision cutting. This time, a bomb was dropped on my ass. I could have fit a softball inside the wound.

In that moment, I believed that I was going to be permanently disfigured. There was no way a human body could recover from that level of damage. I held on to the edge of the bathroom counter. I felt woozy. Every possible worst case scenario burst out of my head. *Did they cut all the way down to my spine? Is my butthole still there? How will I live with half my ass missing? My life is ruined!* The fear overwhelmed me, and I screamed for my mom to come look at it.

She cracked the bathroom door open and asked what I was screaming about. I was scared to show her, and asked her to try not to shout or faint when she saw it. She opened the bathroom door and walked in. I slowly turned around, half-worried that she would lose her mind too. After one glance at it she told me to call 911, or the hospital. Her calm demeanor helped a little, but I knew inside she was screaming too. The previous 2-inch deep wound she had helped me with seemed like nothing more than a scratch compared to this.

I immediately got on the phone and called a number that one of the former in-home nurses had left me. I held back tears as I explained to the person on the line what they did to my body. I am grateful to this day for that mystery customer service person who talked me down from my hysteria, and gave me clear instructions on what to do next.

First, I would have to take a hot shower, as hot as I could bear it, making sure not to get any shampoo or other things into the wound except water. Then, I would need to cover it all up with one big piece of gauze like a blanket, and tape that down. Most importantly, the customer service person scheduled an in-home nurse to arrive later that same day to start doing the gauze changes.

I did as instructed and spent the rest of the day in bed not daring to move an inch. I felt much better when the nurse arrived and saw the wound. She gasped at the size of it. Her shock let me know that this was definitely not normal. The surgeon had literally jacked me up. She had brought her own supplies which we needed since the shoelace type gauze we were going to use wouldn't have been enough to fill in the wound. She used larger square pieces of dressing and pressed them in along the walls of the wound.

Once the first layer was in, she filled in the space with a second layer. Then she covered the outside with a few, very large pieces of gauze, and taped them down. I was glad to have the gauze back in the wound. It felt better than an empty hole. The nurse would end up helping us with the gauze changes for one month. She became a daily visitor and guide throughout the healing process. It was a blessing to have her.

About 2 weeks into the process I had been reading too many

horror stories online about the negative effects of antibiotics, and was scared that they would stop the wound from healing. I stopped taking them without telling anyone, and I really believed I was making a smart move.

Lucky for me the nurse noticed that the wound was looking a bit inflamed during one of her visits. She touched the area that looked concerning, and I felt a bit of pain. She told me the reason it hurt to the touch was because I wasn't taking the medicine. She then lectured me on the importance of taking the pills. If I didn't take them, an infection could grow and prevent the wound from closing. That was enough to get me back on the pills. I started using them again and they fought off any potential infection. The wound didn't hurt to the touch anymore after about two days.

The cavernous opening slowly filled in, almost like a balloon. Within the first month, the left buttcheek healed completely. That was really interesting because after a while I stopped looking at it in the mirror and had no idea that I had regrown that side of my buttcheek until my mom pointed it out to me. The second cheek made slow, but steady, progress throughout the second month. I will give myself some credit because I did not take any painkillers during that whole time. It wasn't painful enough to need them which I thought was great. However, the antibiotics ended up messing my stomach and I spent one Saturday bouncing back and forth between my bedroom and bathroom.

In the final two weeks of healing all that was left was a ping pong sized hole, and the nurse no longer had any home visits scheduled with us. My parents took over and did a great job. They were both getting really good at filling in the wound efficiently without causing me too much discomfort. Around this time I returned to school. It was right before spring break and I made sure to attend enough class sessions to avoid taking a leave of absence. No one noticed that I had a gauze covered wound under my pants.

I also signed up to go on a trip to Mexico with one of my classes for a final project. It would involve a lot of walking and backpacking throughout Mexico City and nearby historical sites. I was worried about damaging the wound, but I didn't want to miss this opportunity and decided to learn how to pack the wound myself. I practiced doing it alone a few times and got pretty good at it.

Before I committed to paying the trip expenses I also wanted to get the doctor's input. At a follow up appointment I asked him if it would be okay for me to travel, and do all the outdoor activities. In his usual manner he brushed aside my concerns and told me that I could even go and ride horses if I wanted to. In his expert opinion nothing would happen and the wound would be fine. I was glad to get cleared, but I didn't like how he seemed to be unbothered by everything. For a moment I considered asking him why he cut out half my ass, but decided there was no point since I was healing up fine. I also figured there was no way a cyst could return after that excision so I would never need to see him or another surgeon for this again.

I went on the trip to Mexico and did the gauze changes myself. It's not too hard as long as you're not icky about pushing gauze into your own body. First I would take a large square piece of gauze and put tape all around the edges. I would lay that on a counter with the sticky side facing up. Then, I would place smaller gauze around the tip of a cue tip and push it into the wound. I had to look backwards using a mirror, but I often felt my way in without using my eyes. Once the cue tip had pushed in the filler gauze, I would pick up the pre-taped gauze from the counter and stick it to the outside of the wound. My friend was staying in a room with me during this trip and he never realized why I took so long in the bathroom after a shower.

For one week, I climbed the pyramids at Teotihuacan, spent hours traveling by bus, hiked up a mountain, and partied late into the night. The gauze stuffed wound never bothered me. There was no pain and I had normal mobility. When I returned to the U.S the entire area soon restored itself into what I like to call "my new ass." All it left was a 6-inch scar. It was incredible. The scar wasn't too bad either, it was like discolored skin with a small dent.

The shocking cyst taught me alot about the amazing ability of the human body to repair itself. I never imagined that I could regrow such a large amount of flesh and skin. It's incredible how the body wants to survive and thrive.

I hope this particular experience didn't freak you out. I think it was an uncommon occurrence resulting from an overzealous surgeon. In fact, a few years later I saw on a local news channel that he was being sued for medical malpractice. I luckily never returned to see this surgeon again.

Based on the amount of flesh he cut out of me, I truly believed that the cyst would never return, but I tried to stay cautious and take proper care of the area. I bought a coccyx cushion again to use on my car seat. Then I started shaving and using No-Bump, an ointment which reduces ingrown hairs and prevents pores from getting clogged. I would shave about once a week using a micro trimmer, instead of a razor, and then would apply the No-Bump.

About two years after this ordeal I felt perfectly fine. I had become a college graduate and was going through rapid life transitions. I was looking to start my career and still trying to find love. Everything seemed to be going great. I felt like I had won the war and little by little stopped taking care of myself again.

First, out went the newest coccyx cushion I had bought. I thought it was annoying to have to sit on it in the car and threw it out. Next, I stopped maintaining the area free of hair and stopped buying No-Bump. I even went back to regular workouts like situps that grinded my tailbone. Finally, I no longer took regular sitting breaks and went back to having bad posture. It was hard to constantly think about a pilonidal and change my daily habits just because it might return. Life was good and I was forgetful.

THE PAINFUL
PILONIDAL

I t came back like a wrecking ball. About 2 years had passed since the shocking pilonidal and I rarely thought about the cyst. One day I began to feel some pressure building up right below the scar. The fear of a recurrence immediately shot into my mind. I tried to take action, but it overwhelmed me before I could do anything to stop it. This was the painful pilonidal.

It sprung up on a relaxing Sunday without any warning. I was hungover and spent most of my day being lazy. I was thinking of getting some junk food and beer to pass the time when out of nowhere, the scar started bothering me. I checked myself in the bathroom mirror and could definitely see that it was looking irritated and a bit swollen. I tried to convince myself that it was a result of sitting with bad posture, and maybe I had even bumped into something.

I started googling my symptoms. I was hoping my search results would reassure me that I just needed to do some warm compress, take a salt bath to relieve the pressure, and stop sitting too much. It's what I looked for, and exactly what I found.

I decided to apply a hot towel to the area to open up my pores and increase ciruclation, but the pressure beneath the scar started to turn into a burning sensation. I quickly prepared a bath with epsom salt and jumped in. After ten minutes of laying in the tub the painful sensation dramatically increased. I was getting desperate for some relief.

I took some Tylenol, got into my car, and drove to a store to buy No-Bump, hoping that it could clear out my pores and do something magical. *Maybe I just have some debris trapped and when the No Bump gets it out I will be fine,* I told myself. Driving back from the store was excruciatingly difficult. I started sweating from fear, and frustration.

With the No-Bump in hand, I rushed into my bathroom, which was now littered with a towel, salt bag, and stale bath water. I opened up the No-Bump bottle and let the liquid fall onto the scar. It flowed down my whole butt and burned my butthole. It didn't help the pain and now my butthole was burning too.

The scar became agonizing. It was inevitable. I knew the cyst was back and trapped under thick scar tissue. If a pilonidal is infected, and can't break through the skin, all the pus and pressure has nowhere to go and might even force its way downward. It was now Sunday night and I was screwed. I knew my local hospital was closed and I decided to take Tylenol and go to bed.

I planned to sleep it off and go see my doctor in the morning if it still bothered me. I was delusional and thought that it might miraculously disappear as long as I didn't sit down. Somehow I fell asleep on my stomach around midnight, most likely because of all the Tylenol.

I woke up to unbearable pain at 7am. Obviously nothing had changed except now I was exhausted from the terrible night of sleep. I immediately got into my can and drove to see my doctor. It was a 15 minute drive of pure agony. When I arrived at the hospital the doors were locked. *Idiot!* I thought. *It's Memorial Day, they aren't open.* As I walked back to my car I needed to start taking baby steps. There was a bag of fluid under my skin and it was ready to pop. Every move I made was beginning to kill me.

I searched for an emergency room on my phone and drove to the nearest one. I drove with my butt off the seat and started sweating. It was now 8am and the place was packed when I entered. I signed in and ended up having to wait the longest two hours of my life. Sitting was impossible, leaning on the wall shot lighting bolts up my back, and walking was pure agony. There was a volcano beneath my tailbone with the pressure building up and nowhere to go.

People kept streaming into the emergency room. Many were in some type of physical pain, and priority was being given to the most urgent cases. As the place filled up I watched one man walk in and stand in line hunched over in pain. He was groaning loudly and holding his arm. He stood in line for at least 2 minutes before one of the front desk attendants called him over, past the other people. I don't know what was wrong with him, but they took him in immediately. I had the strongest urge to start wailing. Maybe someone would move me to the front of the line if I cried loud enough.

The pain was horrific but I couldn't convince myself to fake scream. I continued to watch people arriving and leaving. There was a small room right next to the waiting area with chairs separated by small dividers. Patients were being called into it for the initial analysis and processing. My turn finally came up and by this time I was only able to take very small slow steps. I was directed into the processing room where I took a seat using only my outer buttcheek.

The nurse gathered all my info and took some measurements of my vitals. When I explained what was happening she asked me to point out my pain level on a paper that had different faces expressing emotions. On a scale of 1-10, with 1 being no pain, and 10 being absolutely unberable torture, I chose an 8. I thought it was a reasonable estimate. The nurse sent me back to the waiting area. *Did my pain level determine how quickly I would be seen by a doctor?* I wondered. *Should I have said 10?* Probably not, because I ended up waiting for another 30 minutes while people with the flu, and stuff like that, were moved in ahead of me.

Finally my turn came. A different nurse called my name, and I was directed out of the hospital's entry doors. I thought it was odd. Outside, a doctor was standing next to another patient. Once I finished shuffling out, she lead us towards some bungalows. The doctor was a middle aged, tall, blonde lady with a deeper voice than I expected. She patiently walked alongside me when she saw I was struggling. She was very nice and understanding. I eased my way up a ramp and into the bungalow.

It was larger than it looked from outside, with four examination rooms, and another dreaded waiting area. The other patient was seen before me, leaving me to stand in the waiting room. Nurses kept letting me know that I could take a seat, and I told them that it would be too painful. They didn't need an explanation. In this emergency room they had probably seen a lot. I must have looked a mess too as I was sill semi-hungover, sleep deprived, and very sweaty.

When I finally got my turn in the examination room I laid face down on the bed with my pants down. The doctor knew about pilonidal cyst and recognized what was happening to me immediately. She had worked on pilonidals a few times before and her attending nurse had come across them as well. She touched the scar very gently and I screamed unexpectedly. I was in anguish, and now I was embarrassed too. The doctor confirmed everything that I thought was happening.

"There's a ton of fluid that's trying to get out, it's probably infected, and trying to break through the scar tissue," she explained.

I had figured this out by now and wanted to know what we should do about it.

"It needs to be removed, but in this emergency room we can only do one of two things; I can either send you home with antibiotics, or lance it," she said.

I couldn't believe those were my two options. But to be honest what was I expecting. My mind rummaged through the countless times I didn't take care of myself. This was the end result of my own careless behavior. I could only blame myself and had to deal with the consequences.

In this moment I realized that my unhealthy lifestyle was causing me to fall back under the knife time and again. I took a moment to think about my options. I was still belly down facing away from the doctor. She gave me the time I needed to think. The antibiotics were not likely to work and I couldn't bear the pain any longer. As for the lancing, it would involve cutting through the top layer of scar tissue to release the pressure and drain the cyst. I had seen videos of this online and it looked horrible.

"If you lance it, will the area be numb?" I asked.

"We can't use enough anesthesia to completely numb it." the doctor answered.

"You will have to be fully awake, and feel the whole thing." The nurse added.

She made it very clear what that meant.

"I can give you an injection of local anesthetic, but it will probably not do much, and the lancing will still hurt, a lot." I sensed pity in her voice.

She wanted me to completely understand that there was no avoiding the pain.

Laying on that bed, with tears welling up in my eyes, I shuttered and said, "Let's lance it."

The doctor, her nurse, and I all knew what was coming next. It was going to suck for all of us. The nurse injected a painkiller in my arm that was equal to a few extra strength Tylenol. Next, she brought in a small machine to suck up all the fluids that were going to be released. Then, it was time for a shot of local anesthetic right next to the swelling scar. I laid on my stomach and gripped the frame of the bed as tightly as I could.

The doctor gave me a warning, "Here comes the injection to numb the area, this is going to hurt."

I know it's going to hurt, please stop telling me that, I thought.

Nothing could have prepared me for the absolute agony I would feel. When the injection went in, I screamed and my whole body shook violently. Once the anesthetic was injected the area numbed a bit, but not much. At that point my face was buried into the bed foam, and with clenched teeth, I was tightly gripping the bars on the bed. Tears and sweat were streaming down my face. Nothing but curse words were running through my mind. With the small scalpel in hand, and the nurse ready with the vacuum to suck up the puss, the doctor moved in close. I shut my eyes, gripped harder, clenched harder, and braced for more pain.

"Here comes the cut," the doctor said. "It's going to hurt," she repeated.

Pain, I got it. Just cut me! I cried in my head.

The scalpel sliced into my body and what I felt was life changing. In an odd way it felt like a very spiritual, sort of out of body experience. The cut released a gush of fluid, I let out a loud scream, and the nurse went to work with the suction tube. I screamed and cried for an eternity. The doctor pressed on the scar to force out all the fluid and then, suddenly, I felt nothing except amazing relief.

The volcano had erupted and I was free. She opened the window because apparently the smell was very strong but I was in so much shock that I couldn't smell anything. Once the fluid was cleaned up the doctor and nurse left the room to give me a few minutes to compose myself. I laid there taking deep heavy breaths, exhausted. I was almost able to eek out a small grin as I thought, *it's over, I survived.* I would still need to schedule an excision surgery, but in that moment I was at peace. The nurse came back to clear and sent me on my way. I limped all the way to my car and drove home to figure out how I was going to get another surgery because at that time I wasn't insured.

I was no longer under my parent's health insurance and that was how I covered my previous medical expenses. Since I was working as a tutor, while I tried to find stable work, my only option for health coverage was Obamacare. I went in to see my assigned doctor who informed me that I would need to be put on a waitlist for the surgery. It would take 3-6 months to schedule an operation. That was really difficult to hear. I wanted the pilonidal out of me before the pain returned again. The best he could do for me was prescribe some antibiotics which would run out in about 2 weeks.

Luckily, or I should say through hardwork and determination, I had a great interview with a non-profit and was able to secure a full-time position with health benefits. The medical plan kicked in two weeks later. I started my new position and immediately had to take sick leave. My employer was very understanding of my situation. I was vague about the surgery but let them know I could return within a week. That was a promise I wasn't sure I could keep.

I went back to my original surgeon who I had not seen since the depressing pilonidal a few years back. I trusted his abilities and was glad to be under his care again. And, as a coincidence, the surgery was scheduled the day before Thanksgiving. The excision went great, he left me with a small open wound that my parents and I easily managed without outside help. I made it back to work in the 1 week timeline, but when my supervisor saw me struggling to get through the day she made sure I took extra time to heal up.

After post-operation recovery, I started making positive changes in my life. The painful cyst taught me to take care of myself a lot better and draw strength from my years of experience. It took four pilonidals to finally realize that I can't treat my body like crap and expect different results. I started eating healthier, improving my posture, and making sure to cut back on all the booze and partying. I bought two new coccyx cushions, one for my car, and another for my computer chair. When showering I made sure to wash my hair from back to front and started using a shower glove to keep the cleft free of debris. I was now a full-fledged adult and glad to make long term life changes.

One mistake I made which was hard for me to stop was returning to the gym too quickly. I wanted to exercise and always tried to get back in there as soon as possible. This particular time, soon after my wound had closed up, I actually signed up for personal training sessions. Looking back on it that was a huge mistake and I feel very dumb for doing it. During one training session I was squatting and felt a slight tug within my scar. When I got home I saw speckles of blood from a minor tear in the skin.

That was another big wake up call.

Unfortunately it wasn't until after the next pilonidal that I included a few more essential daily habits to prevent a recurrence, and learned to be more patient.

THE EASY PEASY PILONIDAL

T he 5th and final cyst, so far, was the easiest to manage. When it returned I knew it before the first sign of pain. The fourth cyst was a few years behind me, and it had been almost a decade since the first one. I was very aware of a potential recurrence by this point, and didn't freak out when it happened.

I went back to my original surgeon again, because he always tried to leave me with a manageable wound for a speedy recovery. I believed he would try to do his best work, the least damage to my body, and send me on my way with the proper support. The surgery went well and everything followed the same protocol. The post-op recovery was business as usual and within three weeks my, 1-inch wide and 2-inch deep excision was on its way to being fully healed. This was the easy peasy pilonidal.

My parents were now professionals at wound care and no longer needed the help of an in-home nurse. We had all the necessary equipment and an easy routine to follow. However, I finally gave in and started taking pain killers during my gauze changes. It had been almost 10 years since my first surgery and I was feeling my age. I was no longer the young college student who could bounce back effortlessly. All the cutting and trauma that had taken place over the years had worn me down and I needed the help of pain medication. I was right to be concerned about getting addicted to the pills for all those years because they gave me a nice feeling inside that I started enjoying a little too much.

Luckily, I didn't need them for more than a week because I developed other strategies to help me with pain management. I learned that cussing can increase pain tolerance and I used that to my advantage. During my gauze changes I would pretend that I was being tortured by some enemy to get myself angry, and into fight mode. Then I would spend the time cussing in my head while my parents tended to the wound. This actually worked for me and reduced the pain levels each time.

Another change I made was to start opening up to people close to me about my condition. In the past I always kept up a web of lies and never told anyone outside of my family about what was really going on. I was embarrassed and forced myself to disappear whenever I got treatment and healed.

A close friend finally called me out on it when he told me, "We have no idea where you go, we know something is wrong, but you don't tell us anything." After that I decided to not be ashamed of my condition anymore. I was done lying and hiding the truth. I explained everything to anyone that asked. It was very relieving. I invited people to come visit me and hear about the wound care process. They were all very understanding and wanted the best for me. They liked getting all the gory details, even though it grossed them out. It made the recovery process faster with others being a part of it.

This final cyst was easy to deal with and I was able to use all my previous experiences to get through the entire process with almost no anxiety or fear. I rolled into the hospital like it was another day in the office. I knew the routine and nothing surprised me.

My recovery was much easier as well. I actually turned it into a mini-vacation. I had time to be lazy at home and catch up on shows. Except now I was binge watching shows on Netflix instead of renting DVD's. I made sure to stay away from the gym until weeks after the scar had formed. When I did return, I took it slow with light cardio and built up from there over time.

I made a lot of new changes to my daily habits in order to prevent a recurrence. I believe that these changes are what has kept me healthy for almost 5 years since my fifth pilonidal.

Here are some of the things that I incorporated over the years that are now a regular part of my life. I use a coccyx cushion for just about every chair I sit on, and try to lie down or stand up while watching TV. At work I make sure to use a standing desk as often as possible. I cut back on the drinking and dropped down to a healthier weight. I regularly drink green tea and take vitams for that extra healthy boost.

I also keep the area very clean at all times, even if I am doing something like camping or traveling. I will have a travel pack of supplies, including wipes and baby powder, to keep it clean and prevent moisture buildup. I shower twice a day, washing my hair from back to front to prevent hair from falling towards my butt, and I use a shower glove to scrub inside the crevice. I keep the area free of hair with a micro-trimmer and apply No-Bump afterwards.

Finally, I avoid rolling on my tailbone or any trauma to the area. That's a tough one because I like going to the gym. I have to avoid things like sit ups or heavy lifting while lying down on a workout bench. But I have found ways to work around that issue. With situps I stick to crunches and hanging leg lifts. For bench press, leg press, and other types of presses I focus on balancing over the mid portion of my butt and far away from the tailbone.

It's been a long journey with these little pains in the ass. They have left me with one long scar as a constant reminder of what I have been through. It's about 6 inches long, straight down the cleft of my butt, but it never really bothers me. Sometimes I will get a slight twinge of pain and immediately brace myself for another one to return, but it hasn't happened yet. I treat any sensation from the area very seriously and avoid sitting as much as possible for a few days to give my butt some relief.

When I look back at my first pilonidal, and compare it to the last one, the pain and difficulties are similar, but my perception of them has changed. In the early years a pilonidal would terrify me, leaving me depressed and anxious. Now I perceive it as an opportunity to be on bed rest and take a break. I still get a little scared for what may lie ahead, but overall I feel a lot of positive energy. There may be another one in my future, but until then I plan on enjoying my life. I have been left with an appreciation of my health and determination. The entire experience has made me a much more grateful person.

If you are dealing with pilonidal cyst I hope you admire your own strength and resolve to get through this and give yourself the credit you deserve. Don't lose hope, and don't stop being your badass self. Your internal strength will give you the resolve to thrive and move forward. Never lose that. I also hope you appreciate daily life a little bit more when you get rid of your cyst. It's truly a gift to enjoy a sunny day and take in the beauty of every moment. There are many support groups online where people share tons of personal experiences, check those sites out. They will give you a community to rely on when you're feeling alone.

I now live with my girlfriend who knows that I'm at risk of having another pilonidal, and surgery. I have explained what that means, and how she may need to help me with wound care. She is very ready to give me the support I need. In an interesting twist, she ended up needing an outpatient surgery herself and I was able to help her through the process with all my experience and knowledge. All those surgeries really came in handy.

I have updated this book since I wrote it and will keep doing that regularly as things progress. Hopefully in a few years I can write about a new procedure that completely solves this problem once and for all. Remember to stay strong.

EXCISION SURGERY WALKTHROUGH

The outpatient excision surgery procedure is done in a few hours. Most hospitals follow a similar procedure. Here is a step by step walkthrough.

Pre-Surgery

1. A special soap may be provided to clean bacteria off your skin. This will help prevent the likelihood of an infection during the surgery. If you receive this soap you are to use it the night before your operation and dry yourself with a fresh towel.

2. You may be feeling extremely nervous, anxious, scared or angry that it is happening to you. I find it helpful to imagine the relief that will come from removing the throbbing pain in the ass. It is like an annoying parasite that you will finally destroy.

3. You may not be allowed to eat 8-12 hours before the procedure.

Day Of Surgery

1. You may be required to have someone drive you to the hospital and take you home after the procedure.

2. Wear clothes that are easy to take off and put on such as slippers, shorts, and a baggy shirt. You will want to move as little as possible after the operation.

3. You may be required to arrive at the hospital about 1 or 2 hours before the actual surgery.

4. From the waiting room a nurse will direct you to your hospital bed.

5. This may be the main nurse attending to you during the entire process.

6. You will change out of your clothes and into a hospital gown and socks.

7. They will give you a bag or cubby to put your stuff into. You can usually hold onto your cellphone or anything else you need to keep busy.

8. You will lay down on the hospital bed and continue to wait. The room may be cold, feel free to ask for a blanket.

9. An IV will be inserted into your arm to pump fluids into your body.

10. It may be inserted into your bicep area or the top of your hand.

11. After insertion it can be adjusted, inform the nurse if it hurts too much.

12. It will be taped down to prevent movement of the needle.

13. The anesthesiologist will come in to greet you and explain the process of putting you to sleep.

14. Showtime! You will say goodbye to anyone who came to support, and will be transported on your hospital bed to the operation room.

The Surgery

1. The surgery room will be cold, brightly lit, and full of equipment.

2. There will be a team of people prepping inside.

3. Once you're settled in, the anesthesiologist will put you to sleep. This may happen in different ways:

   a. An oxygen mask is placed over your mouth and nose. You will take deep breaths. The air will feel very cool and pure. Then you will be unconscious.

   b. They will pump some fluid into the IV attached to your arm. You will feel a cold liquid enter your arm. Then you will be unconscious.

Post-Operation

1. You will wake up a few hours later, but it will feel like a few seconds.

2. There will be numbness throughout your body.

3. It will take about 20 minutes before you are able to completely move your body and keep your eyes open.

4. You will feel thirsty, maybe a little sore, but overall tired and sleepy. Water will be provided for you.

5. Your support person will be brought in. You might not be able to talk coherently for about 15 minutes.

6. The nurse will update you on the results and provide instructions for recovery.

7. They will require you to use the bathroom at least once before you are able to go home.

8. You will change back into your regular clothes and head out.

9. Hooray! the toughest part is over.

Recovery

You will no longer have that annoying cyst attached to your body. If you had a painful pilonidal, the area will be numb and feel like there is something missing down there. It is gone and that's what matters. Now comes the time to focus on healing.

Recommendations for open wound care vary, but generally you are required to stuff it with gauze until it fills up from the inside. For closed wounds the area will have stitches and will be sealed up. It requires minimal care and you mostly have to avoid trauma to the area and keep it very clean.

This section will focus on the more complicated open wound recovery.

1. Day one, plan on getting home and doing nothing. Your stomach may be upset or you may have a headache.

2. Day two, you can shower and remove the mounds of medical tape and gauze from the area.

    a. Prepare the gauze, tape, and other supplies that you will need to repack the wound ahead of time.

    b. In the shower, don't be afraid to wash the area with water, but avoid rubbing it, and don't put anything inside the wound. Let the water do the work.

3. Repack gauze into the wound. Lie down and have someone push gauze into the wound until it is filled up.

    a. Make sure they don't use too much or too little gauze. The wound needs to close itself from the bottom first and should be snuggly packed.

    b. After the wound is filled in, cover it with a large piece of gauze and tape that down to hold everything inside.

4. Tips for Packing the wound.

    a. Saline can help clean debris out of the wound. It can be found at most pharmacies.

    b. Use a cue tip to reach the bottom of wounds with smaller entry holes.

    c. There are different sizes of gauze, don't use one that is too large for the wound.

    d. The first time may hurt and feel very strange. If you are sensitive to pain, try taking a painkiller 30 minutes before the gauze change.

c. Find a medical tape that is skin-friendly since you will have to peel it off on a daily basis.

5. First bowel movement. Using the bathroom post-surgery is absolutely doable, but scary. You may experience a mental block. Ease into it slowly and use a counter, or something sturdy, to support your body weight on the way down.

6. Antibiotics may upset your stomach in case you share a bathroom with other's give them a heads up that you may be in there for a while.

7. Try to create a routine and let your body heal. Recovery time will vary depending on the size of your excision, age, and how well you maintain the area. I have healed from open wounds in about 2 weeks to 2 months. Once the wound has fully closed it doesn't mean you are in the clear. I have been foolish enough to hit the gym shortly after healing and caused my wound to tear open from the inside.

The hospital might connect you with a home care agency that can send over a nurse to do the gauze changes every day. For first timers, this can be very helpful since the nurse can teach someone else to do it, and skip past a lot of trial and error.

Prevention

Although I have been unlucky with 5 cysts, I have found that it is often a result of laziness and not taking care of the area. A recurrence is possible years after a surgery, but the chances of it happening can be lowered through preventative actions.

a. Use a coccyx cushion for long periods of sitting.

b. Keep the area free of hair.

c. Wash your hair from back to front to prevent it from falling towards your rear.

d. Use No-Bump after shaving to prevent clogged pores and ingrown hairs.

e. Don't sit with bad posture.

f. Use a shower glove to scrub the area.

g. Shower twice a day.

h. Carry body wipes and baby powder to keep your crevice clean and dry.

i. Wear looser clothing.

j. Avoid situps and other activities that grind or bruise your tailbone.

A Note On Home Remedies

I have used home remedies regularly for pain management and improving my general well being. Warm compress, baths in epsom salt, green tea and turmeric. These things helped alleviate symptoms before the cysts were removed.

a. To do a warm compress I would boil water and pour it on a towel. Then I would lay down and place it over the cyst for 15 minutes a day, twice a day. This would help with the pressure build up in the area.

b. The Epsom salt baths were very relaxing. Epsom salt can be purchased at most local pharmacies. Pour it into your bathtub with warm, or hot water, and immerse yourself in it. The baths helped with destressing and getting blood flow in the area.

c. I started drinking Green tea after my first pilonidal and actually did notice a change in my stomach health. It helped me with a lot of the healing process and side effects of the medications.

d. I tried turmeric as a pill supplement and in powder form to add to my tea. It apparently helps with symptoms of pilonidal cyst, but I can't say I noticed a difference other than a placebo effect.

REFERENCES

Aithal, S. K., Rajan, C.S., & Reddy, N. (2012). Limberg Flap for Saccrococcygeal Pilonidal Sinus a safe and sound procedure. Indian Journal of Surgery, 75(4), 298-301. doi:10.1007/s12262-012-0489-5

Bali, I., Aziret, M., Sozen, S., Emir, S., Erdem, H., Cetinkunar, S., & Irkorucu, O. (2015). Effectiveness of Limberg and Karydakis flap in recurrent pilonidal sinus disease. Clinics, 70(5), 350-355. doi:10.6061/clinics/2015(05)08

Fahrni, G.T., Vuille-Dit-Bille, R.N., Leus, S., Meuli, M., Staerkle, R.F., Fink, L., Dincler, S., Muff, B. S. (2016). Five-year follow up and recurrence rates following surgery for acute and chronic pilonidal disease: A survey of 421 cases. Wounds, 28(1).

Hosseini, S. V., Bananzadeh, A. M., Rivaz, M., Sabet, B., Mosallae, M., Pourahmad, S., & Yarmohammadi, H. (2006). The comparison between drainage, delayed excision and primary closure with excision and secondary healing in management of pilonidal abscess. International Journal of Surgery, 4(4), 228-231. doi: 10.1016/j.ijsu.2005.12.005

Jain, A., & Thambuchetty, N. (2016). Management of pilonidal sinus disease: A 5 years retrospective

analysis. International Surgery Journal, 586-588. doi:

10.18203/2349-2902.isj20161127

Pappas, A. F., & Christodoulou, D.K. (2018). A new minimally invasive treatment of pilonidal sinus disease with the use of a diode laser.: A prospective large series of patients. Colorectal Disease, 20(8). doi: 10.1111/codi.14285

Stauffer, V. K., Luedi, M., Kauf, P., Schmid, M., Diekmann, M., Wieferich, K., Schnuriger, B., Doll, D. (2018). Common surgical procedures in pilonidal sinus disease: A meta-analysis, merged data analysis, and comprehensive study on recurrence. Scientific Reports, 8(1). doi: 10.1038/s41598-018-20143-4

Yoldas, T., Karaca, C., Unalp, O., Uguz, A., Caliskan, C., Akgun, E., & Korkut, M. (2013). Recurrent pilonidal sinus: Lay open or flap closure, does it differ? International Surgery, 98(4), 319-323. doi:10.9738/intsurg-d-13-00081.1

www.ingramcontent.com/pod-product-compliance
Lightning Source LLC
Chambersburg PA
CBHW030716220526
45463CB00005B/2065